Diversity, Equity, and Inclusion in Hand Surgery

Editors

MICHAEL G. GALVEZ
KEVIN C. CHUNG

HAND CLINICS

www.hand.theclinics.com

Consulting Editor
KEVIN C. CHUNG

February 2023 • Volume 39 • Number 1

ELSEVIER

1600 John F. Kennedy Boulevard • Suite 1800 • Philadelphia, Pennsylvania, 19103-2899

http://www.theclinics.com

HAND CLINICS Volume 39, Number 1
February 2023 ISSN 0749-0712, ISBN-13: 978-0-323-93873-0

Editor: Megan Ashdown
Developmental Editor: Hannah Almira Lopez

Hand Clinics (ISSN 0749-0712) is published quarterly by Elsevier Inc., 360 Park Avenue South, New York, NY 10010-1710. Months of publication are February, May, August, and November. Business and Editorial Offices: 1600 John F. Kennedy Blvd., Ste. 1800, Philadelphia, PA 19103-2899. Customer Service Office: 3251 Riverport Lane, Maryland Heights, MO 63043. Periodicals postage paid at New York, NY and at additional mailing offices. Subscription price is $444.00 per year (domestic individuals), $878.00 per year (domestic institutions), $100.00 per year (domestic students/residents), $506.00 per year (Canadian individuals), $1023.00 per year (Canadian institutions), $568.00 per year (international individuals), $1023.00 per year (international institutions), $256.00 (international students/residents), and $100.00 (Canadian students/residents). Foreign air speed delivery is included in all *Clinics* subscription prices. All prices are subject to change without notice. **POSTMASTER:** Send address changes to *Hand Clinics*, Elsevier Health Sciences Division, Subscription Customer Service, 3251 Riverport Lane, Maryland Heights, MO 63043. Customer Service (orders, claims, online, change of address): Elsevier Health Sciences Division, Subscription **Customer Service, 3251 Riverport Lane, Maryland Heights, MO 63043. Tel: 1-800-654-2452 (U.S. and Canada); 314-447-8871 (outside U.S. and Canada). Fax: 314-447-8029. E-mail: journalscustomerservice-usa@elsevier.com (for print support); journalsonlinesupport-usa@elsevier.com (for online support).**

Reprints. For copies of 100 or more of articles in this publication, please contact the Commercial Reprints Department, Elsevier Inc., 360 Park Avenue South, New York, New York 10010-1710. Tel.: 212-633-3874; Fax: 212-633-3820; E-mail: reprints@elsevier.com.

Hand Clinics is covered in *MEDLINE/PubMed (Index Medicus), Current Contents/Clinical Medicine, EMBASE/Excerpta Medica,* and *ISI/BIOMED.*

Contributors

CONSULTING EDITOR

KEVIN C. CHUNG, MD, MS
Charles B.G. de Nancrede Professor of Surgery, Professor of Plastic Surgery and Orthopaedic Surgery, Chief of Hand Surgery, Department of Surgery, Section of Plastic Surgery, Michigan Medicine, Assistant Dean for Faculty Affairs, Associate Director of Global REACH, University of Michigan Medical School, Comprehensive Hand Center, University of Michigan, The University of Michigan Health System, Ann Arbor, Michigan

EDITORS

MICHAEL G. GALVEZ, MD
Pediatric Hand and Upper Extremity Surgery, Division of Plastic and Hand Surgery, Valley Children's Healthcare, Madera, California

KEVIN C. CHUNG, MD, MS
Charles B.G. de Nancrede Professor of Surgery, Professor of Plastic Surgery and Orthopaedic Surgery, Chief of Hand Surgery, Department of Surgery, Section of Plastic Surgery, Michigan Medicine, Assistant Dean for Faculty Affairs, Associate Director of Global REACH, University of Michigan Medical School, Comprehensive Hand Center, University of Michigan, The University of Michigan Health System, Ann Arbor, Michigan

AUTHORS

MARK BARATZ, MD
Department of Orthopaedics, University of Pittsburgh Medical Center, Bethel Park, Pennsylvania

CHRISTOPHER O. BAYNE, MD
Chief, Hand, Upper Extremity, and Microvascular Surgery, Department of Orthopaedic Surgery, University of California, Davis, Sacramento, California

BRITTANY BEHAR, MD
Associate Professor, Department of Plastic/Maxillofacial Surgery, University of Virginia, Charlottesville, Virginia

LAXMINARAYAN BHANDARI, MCH
Hand Surgeon, Kleinert Kutz Associates, Louisville, Kentucky

CATHLEEN CAHILL, MD
Orthopaedic Surgery Resident, UChicago Medicine and Biological Sciences, Chicago, Illinois

WENDY CHEN, MD, MS
Assistant Professor, University of Texas at Houston McGovern Medical School, Houston, Texas

A. BOBBY CHHABRA, MD
Lillian T. Pratt Distinguished Professor and Chair of Orthopaedic Surgery, Department of Orthopaedic Surgery, Hand Surgery, University of Virginia Health, Charlottesville, Virginia

KEVIN C. CHUNG, MD, MS
Charles B.G. de Nancrede Professor of Surgery, Professor of Plastic Surgery and

Orthopaedic Surgery, Chief of Hand Surgery, Department of Surgery, Section of Plastic Surgery, Michigan Medicine, Assistant Dean for Faculty Affairs, Associate Director of Global REACH, University of Michigan Medical School, Comprehensive Hand Center, University of Michigan, The University of Michigan Health System, Ann Arbor, Michigan

KELLY BETTINA CURRIE, MD
Department of Surgery, Division of Plastic and Reconstructive Surgery, Washington University in St. Louis School of Medicine, St Louis, Missouri

JENNIFER D'AURIA, MD
Department of Orthopaedics, University of Pittsburgh Medical Center, Bethel Park, Pennsylvania

ANGELO R. DACUS, MD
Professor, Vice Chair for Diversity, Inclusion and Wellness, Department of Orthopaedic Surgery, University of Virginia, Charlottesville, Virginia

MARVIN DINGLE, MD
OrthoCarolina Hand and Upper Extremity Fellow 2022-2023, Assistant Professor, Department of Surgery, Uniformed Services University of Health Sciences, Walter Reed National Military Medical Center, Bethesda, Maryland

CLAIRE A. DONNELLEY, MD
Department of Orthopaedics and Rehabilitation, Yale University, New Haven, Connecticut

MICHAEL G. GALVEZ, MD
Pediatric Hand and Upper Extremity Surgery, Division of Plastic and Hand Surgery, Valley Children's Healthcare, Madera, California

ANDREA HALIM, MD
Department of Orthopaedics and Rehabilitation, Yale University, New Haven, Connecticut

MARIA T. HUAYLLANI, MD
Department of Plastic and Reconstructive Surgery, The Ohio State University Wexner Medical Center, Columbus, Ohio

LISA L. LATTANZA, MD, FAOA, FAAOS
Professor of Orthopaedics and Rehabilitation, Chair, Orthopaedics and Rehabilitation, Chief, Yale New Haven Hospital, Department of Orthopaedics and Rehabilitation, Yale University, New Haven, Connecticut

HANNAH LEE, MD
Department of Orthopaedics, University of Pittsburgh Medical Center, Pennsylvania

JOSEPH PAUL LETZELTER, MD
Assistant Professor, Orthopaedic Surgery Department, Children's National Medical Center, Washington, DC

MEGAN CONTI MICA, MD
Associate Professor of Orthopaedic Surgery and Rehabilitation Medicine, UChicago Medicine and Biological Sciences, Chicago, Illinois

AMY M. MOORE, MD
Professor and Chair, Department of Plastic and Reconstructive Surgery, The Ohio State University Wexner Medical Center, Columbus, Illinois

PAIGE L. MYERS, MD
Assistant Professor, Department of Surgery, Section of Plastic Surgery, University of Michigan, Ann Arbor, Michigan

UZAIR QAZI, MD
Burn Surgery Fellow, Indiana University School of Medicine, Indianapolis, Indiana

SHEA RAY, MD, MS
Department of Orthopaedics, University of Pittsburgh Medical Center, Bethel Park, Pennsylvania

TIAM M. SAFFARI, MD, PhD, MSc
Department of Plastic and Reconstructive Surgery, The Ohio State University Wexner Medical Center, Columbus, Ohio

JULIE BALCH SAMORA, MD, PhD, MPH, FAAOS, FAOA
Medical Director of Safety, Orthopaedic Surgery, Nationwide Children's Hospital, Columbus, Ohio

MICAH K. SINCLAIR, MD
Department of Orthopaedic Surgery and Musculoskeletal Medicine, Children's Mercy

Hospital, Associate Professor, University of Missouri Kansas City, Education Assistant Professor, University of Kansas Medical Center, Kansas City, Missouri

KASHYAP KOMARRAJU TADISINA, MD
Department of Surgery, Division of Plastic and Reconstructive Surgery, Washington University in St. Louis School of Medicine, St Louis, Missouri

ERICA TAYLOR, MD, MBA
Orthopaedic Hand Surgeon, Associate Chief Medical Officer for DEI, Duke Health Physician Organization, Founder, Orthopaedic Diversity Leadership Consortium, Duke University School of Medicine

KAMALI THOMPSON, MD, MBA
Temple University Hospital, Philadelphia, Pennsylvania

ALLYNE TOPAZ, MD
Resident Physician, University of Texas Medical Branch at Galveston, Galveston, Texas

KIA WASHINGTON, MD
Division of Plastic and Reconstructive Surgery, Professor, University of Colorado, Aurora, Colorado

Contents

Preface: The Value of Diversity: Spectrum of Tissue, Training, and Individuals in Hand Surgery xiii

Michael G. Galvez and Kevin C. Chung

Diverse Leadership in Hand Surgery: Foundation on the Shoulder of Giants 1

Tiam M. Saffari, Maria T. Huayllani, and Amy M. Moore

Surgical leaders exhibit unique characteristics that allow them to impact and innovate their respective fields. In Hand Surgery, we recognize areas of leadership success, including leadership of position, leadership of innovation, and academic leadership. This article aims to define the term "success" and provide examples of how a diverse climate can lead to leadership success by highlighting a few stories of diverse giants in the field of Hand Surgery.

The Value of Diversity, Equity, and Inclusion: Race and Ethnicity Affecting Patients 9

Christopher O. Bayne

Patient race and ethnicity are important factors in health-care inequity, including care for the patient with hand and upper extremity pathologic condition. Physician diversity has been shown to promote better access, improve health-care quality, and improve satisfaction for underserved populations. Concordance, most often defined as a similarity or shared identity between physician and patient, has been shown to have a positive influence on health-care disparities. Although diversity among Hand surgeons is increasing, it is not matching the diversity of the population as a whole. It is imperative that we work to increase and maintain diversiARty in order to provide the best care for our patients.

Role of Health Equity Research and Policy for Diverse Populations Requiring Hand Surgery Care 17

Paige L. Myers and Kevin C. Chung

Health equity requires allocation of resources to eliminate the systematic disparities in health, imposed on marginalized groups, which adversely impact outcomes. A socioecological approach is implemented to elucidate the role of health equity research and policy for underrepresented minority and socioeconomically disadvantaged populations. Through investigation of the individual, community, institution, and public policy, we investigate problems and propose solutions to ensure fair and just treatment of all patients requiring hand surgery.

Advocacy for Diversity in Hand Surgery 25

Angelo R. Dacus, Brittany Behar, and Kia Washington

Diversity in the Hand Surgery workforce improves the quality of care delivered, advances a wider variety of innovation within the field and leads to higher patient satisfaction, greater access to care and patient adherence to advice. An understanding of the data makes a compelling argument for change. Advocacy is necessary to stop the "leaky pipeline" of the loss of diversity in more senior and leadership roles. Hand surgeons who are both women and from underrepresented minority groups are especially vulnerable to bias from the health-care system, with focused support and mentoring required throughout their training and career.

difficult but not impossible. A comprehensive strategy for an UIM student to become a hand surgeon is outlined in detail.

LGBTQ+ Perspective in Hand Surgery: Surgeon and Patient **79**

Joseph Paul Letzelter and Julie Balch Samora

Lesbian, gay, bisexual, transgender, queer, and other sexual and gender minority (LGBTQ+) individuals and patients face high levels of discrimination both in the workplace and in the clinic setting, with more than 25% of LGBTQ+ people experiencing discrimination in the workplace due to their sexual orientation. Hand Surgery stands to continue to advance by encouraging the brightest students into the field no matter their background. LGBTQ+ patients also have specific needs within the field of Hand Surgery, where we are uniquely positioned to treat them or guide them by being well versed in the needs of the community.

The International Medical Graduate Perspective in Hand Surgery: Legacy and Future Challenges **87**

Uzair Qazi and Laxminarayan Bhandari

International medical graduates (IMGs) have made significant contributions in the field of hand surgery in terms of bringing in skill, innovation, research, and leadership and have gone onto mentor the next generations of hand surgeons. In this article, we have highlights some such contributions. We also highlight various pathways that IMGs take to establish their practice in the United States and the various challenges and hurdles they face.

Microaggressions and Implicit Bias in Hand Surgery **95**

Kashyap Komarraju Tadisina and Kelly Bettina Currie

Implicit bias and microaggressions are well-known phenomenon and have recently been acknowledged as contributing to health care disparities. Within Hand Surgery, implicit bias and microaggressions occur in patient-surgeon, surgeon-peer, surgeon-staff, and training environment interactions. Although racial and gender biases are well studied, biases can also be based on age, sexual orientation, socioeconomic background, and/or hierarchal rank. Academia has well-documented evidence of implicit bias and microaggressions, contributing to current disparate demographics of trainees, physicians, and leaders within Hand Surgery. Awareness is fundamental to combating bias and microaggressions; however, actions must be taken to minimize negative effects and change culture.

Allyship for Diversity, Equity, and Inclusion in Hand Surgery **103**

Shea Ray, Jennifer D'Auria, Hannah Lee, and Mark Baratz

This article endeavors to be a resource to those individuals interested in becoming an ally or educating potential allies in the field of Hand Surgery. The definitions of allyship, its history, and its expected benefits are considered. The qualities of a good ally are enumerated, and approaches to becoming a better ally are described. The authors provide personal experience with impactful allies and describe strategies and resources on a local and national level. The authors conclude with "Bigger Questions": those issues that seem essential to have allyship succeed in expanding diversity, equity, and inclusion in the specialty.

Recruitment of the Next Generation of Diverse Hand Surgeons **111**

Claire A. Donnelley, Andrea Halim, and Lisa L. Lattanza

Hand surgery encompasses a diaspora of pathology and patients, but the surgeons treating this population are not commensurately diverse. A physician population that

reflects the population it treats consistently leads to improved patient outcomes. Despite increasing diversity amongst surgeons entering into pipeline specialties such as General Surgery, Plastic Surgery, and Orthopaedic Surgery, the overall makeup of practicing hand surgeons remains largely homogenous. This article outlines organizations, such as the Perry Initiative, which have increased recruitment of women and underrepresented minorities into pipeline programs. Techniques of minimizing bias and increasing opportunities for underrepresented groups are also discussed.

HAND CLINICS

FORTHCOMING ISSUES

May 2023
Current Concepts in Flexor Tendon Repair and Rehabilitation
Rowena McBeath and Kevin Chung, *Editors*

August 2023
Managing Difficult Problems in Hand Surgery: Challenges, Complications and Revisions
Sonu Jain, *Editor*

November 2023
Innovation in Upper Extremity Fracture Treatment
Lauren M. Shapiro and Robin N. Kamal, *Editors*

RECENT ISSUES

November 2022
Avascular Necrosis of the Carpal Bones: Etiologies and Treatments
Mitchell Pet and Charles Andrew Daly, *Editors*

August 2022
Challenging Current Wisdom in Hand Surgery
Jin Bo Tang and Grey Giddins, *Editors*

May 2022
Current Concepts in Thumb Carpometacarpal Joint Disorders
Phillip Ross and Sarah Sasor, *Editors*

Preface

The Value of Diversity: Spectrum of Tissue, Training, and Individuals in Hand Surgery

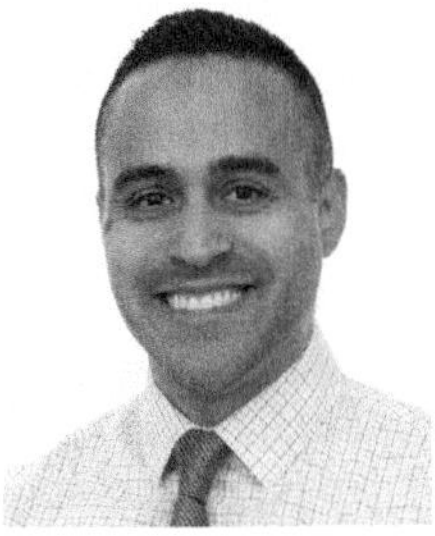
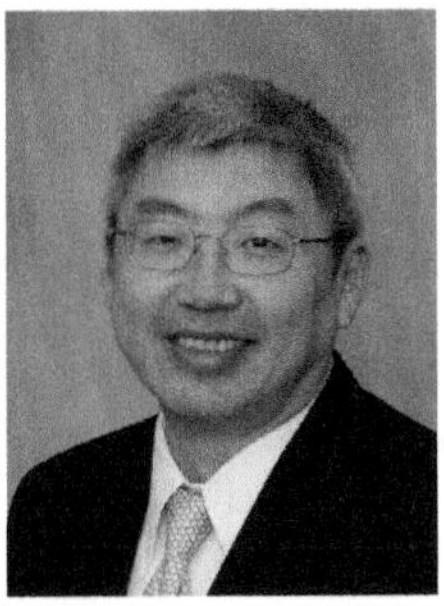

Michael G. Galvez, MD Kevin C. Chung, MD, MS
Editors

> *"It falls to few men to originate a surgical specialty."*
>
> *— Sterling Bunnell*

The field of Hand Surgery was founded by Dr Sterling Bunnell, who was asked by the US Surgeon General, during World War II, to develop regional hand centers at Army Hospitals in the United States. The history of the founding of Hand Surgery is important knowledge. The "few men" were the founders of the field and included only White men (**Fig. 1**). Dr Bunnell believed that Hand Surgery was a "composite problem requiring the correlation of the various specialties—Orthopaedic, Plastic and Neurologic Surgery—the knowledge of any one of which alone is inadequate for repairing the hand." This concept of bringing together several surgical specialties becomes essential to take care of all the tissues of the hand and upper extremity to repair and reconstruct all the necessary structures in a coordinated fashion.

Diversity, equity, and inclusion may be a topic that seems irrelevant to the field of hand and upper extremity. However, with close attention, there is a significant correlation. To become a hand and upper-extremity surgeon, one must either complete an Orthopedic, Plastic, or General Surgery residency and then complete an additional one-year fellowship in hand and upper extremity. We are all aware the foundation of training in Hand Surgery is based upon the amount of Hand Surgery that was experienced in residency. This can be incredibly different experiences depending on the training program. There is significant variability in Hand Surgery fellowships with the breadth of Hand Surgery performed (from shoulder to fingertip), which can include shoulder, elbow, forearm, distal radius, wrist, congenital hand differences, microsurgery, replantation, complex reconstruction, and so on. This variability in training and interests results in variable types of practices. Orthopaedic Hand surgeons can sometimes be less comfortable with microsurgery and therefore less likely to perform. Plastic Hand surgeons can sometimes be less comfortable with complex distal radius and forearm injuries and less likely to perform them. When we think about Hand Surgery, this field combines all these levels of expertise with our ability to change form and anatomy, change function, and use technology such as the microscope and hardware to best reconstruct the diverse tissue of the upper extremity. As Hand surgeons, we clearly value the diversity of pathways for training so that we can consider all the tissues when performing reconstruction.

In a similar fashion, we should value the diversity of who is being trained to become a Hand surgeon. Why should we care? Because diversity in the physician/surgeon workforce has been shown to improve patient outcomes. The disparity in

Hand Clin 39 (2023) xiii–xv
https://doi.org/10.1016/j.hcl.2022.08.010

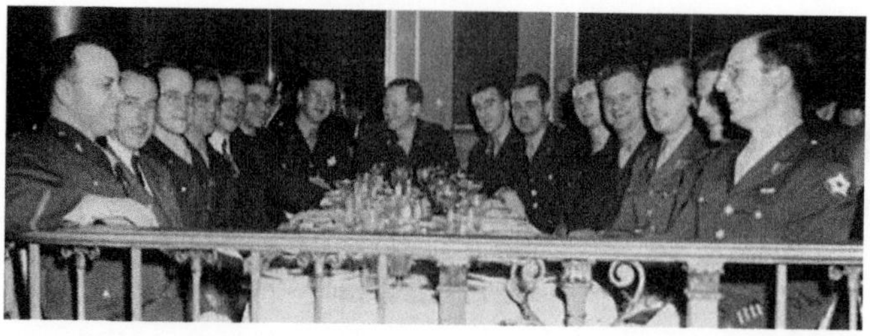

Fig. 1. Founding members image on ASSH.org. (*Courtesy of* the American Society for Surgery of the Hand, Chicago, IL; with permission)

health care access and outcomes across the United States has been made readily apparent during the COVID-19 pandemic. In Hand Surgery, the number of women entering the field has increased over time, although remains low, and the number of underrepresented minorities have remained persistently low. Hand surgeons of the United States should reflect the diversity of our populations. We have disparity in the access for Hand surgeons in the United States; therefore, we should be working on recruiting the next generation of Hand Surgeons that are, it is hoped, more likely to work within their own community to help close these gaps.

We are excited to provide you with this series of thoughtful articles by Hand Surgery leaders on crucial topics within diversity, equity, and inclusion. Our history becomes incredibly important and includes many contributions from Hand surgeons from diverse backgrounds. Our diverse patient populations come from different demographics, ethnicity, and race, whose outcomes are affected. Research in health equity and policy is important for understanding where to improve outcomes. We value having Hand surgeons from diverse backgrounds, including race, ethnicity, sex, and sexual orientation, which clearly drives excellence. Improving diversity comes from the top, from our leadership, and therefore, it becomes important to have a sustainable approach in improving diversity within academics and the community. Success in this subspecialized field requires mentorship and sponsorship, with the goals of aligning this topic for the mentee. Women have made significant contributions to the field over time, and there are important considerations that must be considered for a supportive environment in Hand Surgery. The underrepresented minority is rare in Hand Surgery, and the goal should be to make them commonplace. The LGBTQ+ experience within Hand Surgery for surgeons and patients is also an important consideration for inclusivity. The international medical graduate perspective, both historical and challenges, has never been openly discussed before within the field of Hand Surgery. To survive training and practice, microaggressions and implicit bias are important considerations for many. Our leaders serve as allies and advocates for those that come from diverse backgrounds,

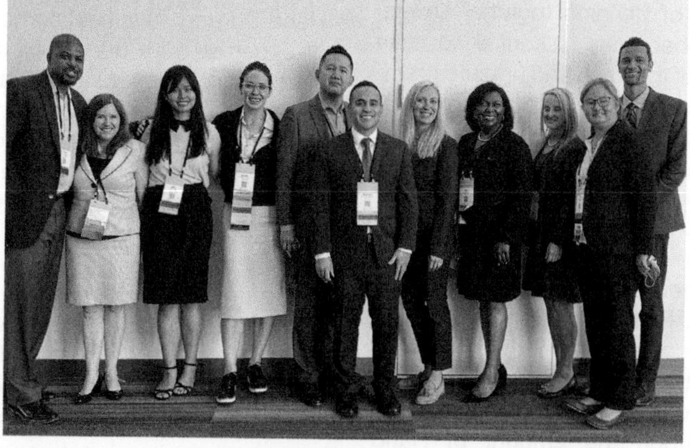

Fig. 2. Committed individuals, from diverse backgrounds, continuing and expanding excellence in the subspecialty of hand and upper-extremity surgery. (*Courtesy of* Michael Galvez, MD, Madera, CA)

and their support is essential. Finally, we must focus on medical students and residents for the recruitment and retention of the next generation of diverse Hand surgeons. We are proud of these essential topics that deserve a presence within our literature.

An active and concerted multifaceted approach will foster change. We respect and honor the founders of our society, but it is time to implement diversity and advocate for allowing others to sit at the table (**Fig. 2**) and contribute, with the hopes of better reflecting our diverse patient populations of the United States. We hope that you enjoy this issue and can take the information, the data, and the drive, and join us in taking action and moving our field *forward*.

"*It falls to many committed individuals, from diverse backgrounds, to continue and expand excellence in the subspeciality of hand and upper-extremity surgery*."

Michael G. Galvez, MD
Pediatric Hand and Upper Extremity Surgery
Division of Plastic and Hand Surgery
Valley Children's Healthcare
9300 Valley Children's Place GE07
Madera, CA 93636, USA

Kevin C. Chung, MD, MS
Section of Plastic Surgery
Department of Surgery, University of Michigan
2130 Taubman Center
1500 East Medical Center Drive
Ann Arbor, MI 48109, USA

E-mail addresses:
michaelgalvez@gmail.com (M.G. Galvez)
kecchung@med.umich.edu (K.C. Chung)

Diverse Leadership in Hand Surgery

Foundation on the Shoulder of Giants

Tiam M. Saffari, MD, PhD, MSc[a], Maria T. Huayllani, MD[a],
Amy M. Moore, MD[b,*]

KEYWORDS

• Diversity • Equity • Leadership • Success • Hand surgery

KEY POINTS

- Defining success is different for each individual and is defined in different areas of life.
- Being successful is not just talent, but encompasses passion and perseverance for long-term goals (ie, grit).
- Leadership of position, leadership of innovation, and academic leadership are the types of leadership held by our diverse giants in Hand Surgery.
- Diversification of our leaders will follow efforts to increase diversity within our field.

BACKGROUND

Leaders in the field of surgery exhibit unique characteristics that qualify them to impact and innovate their respective fields. James McGregor Burns wrote in 1978 that "*leadership is one of the most observed and least understood phenomena on earth.*"[1] Evolutionarily, a leader-follower relationship naturally develops when a group of people come together, recognizing leadership as a universal human behavior.[2,3] Goleman, Boyatzis, and McKee[4] described followership as the mirror image of leadership, and it is widely recognized that one does not exist without the other. Traditionally, positions of leadership have not been diverse. In medicine, like most disciplines, leadership opportunities have been fulfilled by White men.[5,6] This fact is neither to diminish the importance of such leaders nor take away their success, but allows us to examine our own specialty and identify trends. More importantly, we aimed to look at those few diverse leaders that have arisen in Hand Surgery and to try to identify commonalities among them (**Fig. 1**).

With 19% of women, Hand Surgery represents one of the highest female rates among plastic and orthopedic surgery subspecialties.[7] Although this percentage has been increasing in medicine, representation of women in leadership positions has been lagging, a phenomenon called "the leaky pipeline."[8,9] From 2012 to 2021, surgical society presidents were found to be predominantly White (87.6%) and male (83.4%).[6] Only 2 of the 121 combined presidents of American Association for Hand Surgery (AAHS) and American Society for Surgery of the Hand (ASSH) (1.7%) have been female (ie, Susan Mackinnon and Marybeth Ezaki, respectively) and women have held only 12 of 96 (12.5%) of council positions.[10] Similarly, there has been a marked increase in the diversity of the US population without this being reflected in the field of Hand Surgery. An increase in representation of less than 1% per year has been reported for African Americans, Hispanics, Asians, and females in Hand Surgery, and there is still an underrepresentation among all trainees.[11]

Despite the disparities found within Hand Surgery leadership, our field has had multiple diverse

[a] Department of Plastic and Reconstructive Surgery, The Ohio State University Wexner Medical Center, Columbus, OH, USA; [b] Department of Plastic and Reconstructive Surgery, The Ohio State University Wexner Medical Center, 915 Olentangy River Road, Suite 2100, Columbus, IL 43212, USA
* Corresponding author.
E-mail address: amy.m.moore@osumc.edu

Hand Clin 39 (2023) 1–8
https://doi.org/10.1016/j.hcl.2022.08.023
0749-0712/23/

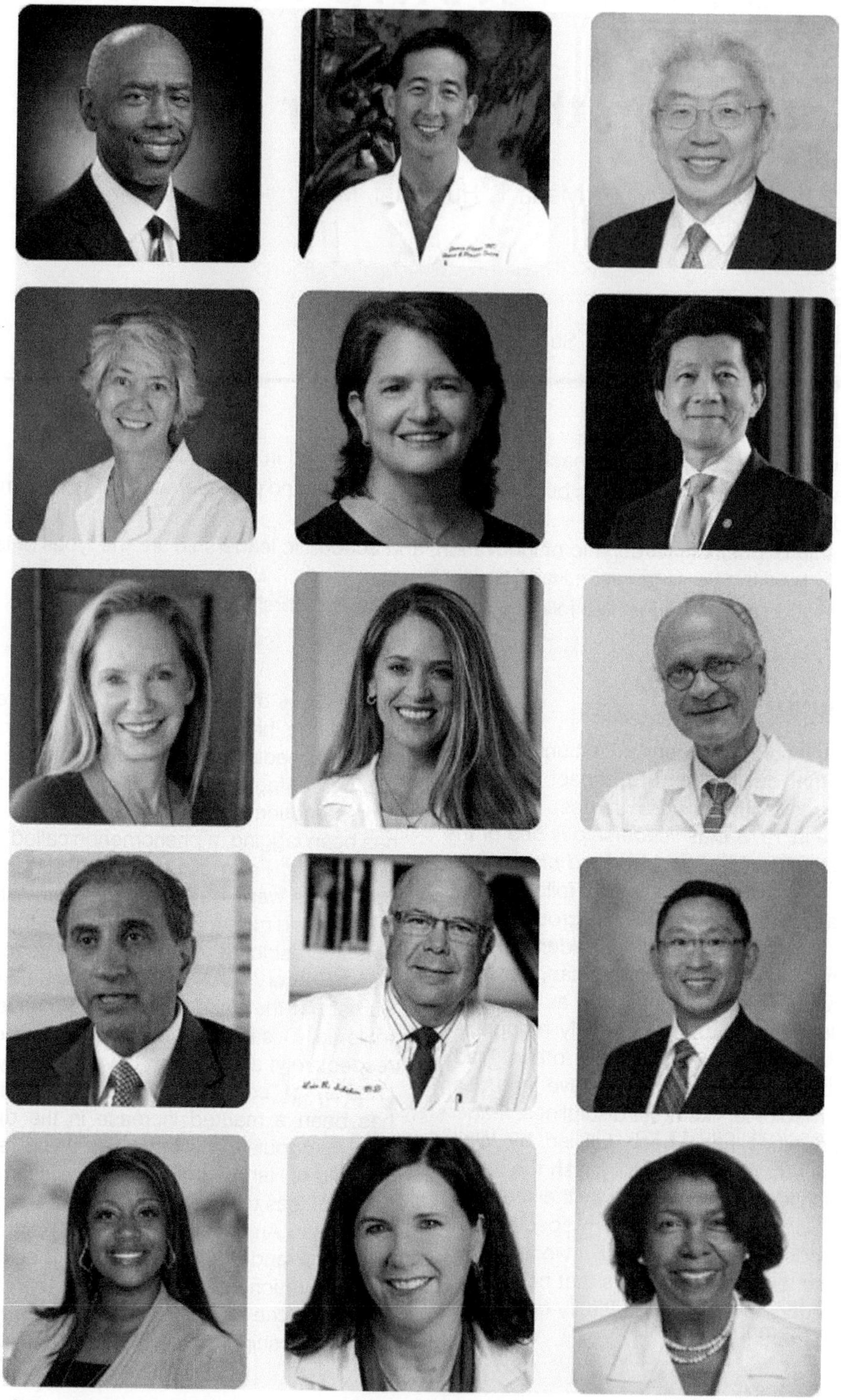

Fig. 1. Our diverse leaders in Hand Surgery. From left to right (in alphabetical order): Dr Milton Armstrong, Dr James Chang, Dr Kevin Chung, Dr Marybeth Ezaki, Dr Lisa Lattanza, Dr W.P. Andrew Lee, Dr Susan E. Mackinnon, Dr Amy M. Moore, Dr Jorge L. Orbay, Dr Ghazi M. Rayan, Dr Luis Scheker, Dr Alexander Shin, Dr Erica Taylor, Dr Jennifer M. Wolf, and Dr Kerri Woodberry.

leaders who have had significant success and provide a face for the future. This article recognizes areas of leadership success including leadership of position, leadership of innovation, and academic leadership. Although not all inclusive, the article provides examples of how a diverse climate can lead to leadership success by highlighting a few stories of diverse giants in Hand Surgery.

How to Define Success

Many, including Maya Angelou, believe that "success" is about enjoying your work. As an American poet and civil rights activist, Angelou mentions that "*success is liking yourself, liking what you do, and liking how you do it.*" In a society that is driven by numbers, it is nearly impossible to not have a set definition of success. Are you successful when having published 100 papers or received 5 grants or do we define success by having achieved a leadership position? Defining "success" is different for each individual and defined in different areas of life (ie, emotional success, financial success, professional success). Many agree that success as a general term is "the achievement of a desired goal." Dr Susan Mackinnon, a pioneer in nerve surgery and the first female president of the AAHS, defines professional success as "leading a purposeful and powerful life" and personal success as "loving others and being loved." Success is achieved by perseverance in failure, beautifully captured by the Japanese proverb "Fall down seven times, stand up eight."

The concept of resilience and embracing failure is recognized by many leaders in our field of Hand Surgery, including Dr Alexander Shin, an orthopedic brachial plexus and hand surgeon who served as the hand fellowship director for 9 years at Mayo Clinic (2008–2017, Rochester, MN, USA). He reports that experiencing failure pushes you to find other routes that lead to your desired goal; this eventually leads to success. Dr Mackinnon also recognizes failure as one of the factors to become successful. "Failure must be identified, embraced and we must learn from it." Other factors contributing to success that have been mentioned in her 2013 TEDx talk are having good mentors and collaborators, serendipity, and working hard for a long period.

Being successful is not just talent, but encompasses passion and perseverance for long-term goals, or termed "grit" by Angela Duckworth. Grit is defined by 5 characteristics: courage, conscientiousness, perseverance, resilience, and passion.[12] Interestingly, grit does not correlate with intelligence quotient (IQ). Incremental predictive validity of success measures over and beyond IQ and conscientiousness. Collectively, it was found that the achievement of difficult goals entails not only entail talent but also a sustained and focused application of talent over a long period.[12] The senior author is a firm believer of this concept and attributes "grit" to her success. Achieving the position of Chair and Professor in Plastic Surgery (The Ohio State University, Columbus, OH, USA) within 10 years of completing residency, Dr Moore mentions that "the definition of success can vary on a daily basis, but must be defined by oneself - not by others." Success for Dr Moore is ever-changing. It is "curing someone's pain with a surgical procedure, getting the next grant funded, hiring the next new faculty, retaining her current faculty, making it to her children's activities and remembering her loved ones' birthdays." We encourage the next generation, our future leaders, to focus on what brings you joy because we believe "if you love what you do, and do what you love, success will follow."

How a Diverse Climate Would Benefit Success

Diversity serves as an umbrella term to characterize various dimensions of heterogeneity, that is, gender, nationality, ethnic origin, religion or worldview, disability, age, sexual orientation, and identity.[13] Having a diverse team allows for increased sets of skills compared with homogeneous groups, aiding in enhanced ability to problem solving. A causative link has been found between the innovation of a company and their diverse workforce.[14] It has been suggested that innovation comes from freedom of thought and interaction with others, a factor that is supported in a diverse environment. Dr Milton Armstrong, hand surgeon and Chief of Plastic Surgery at the Medical University of South Carolina in Charleston, is an accomplished leader and educator. He came from humble origins and was the first of his family to pursue a career in medicine. Despite the difficulties he encountered, he completed his general surgery residency, plastic and reconstructive surgery residency, and Hand Surgery fellowship. Perhaps the constant work, motivation (ie, grit), and having great support made the difference in succeeding. As Chief, Dr Armstrong is committed to providing strong leadership, guidance, and an innovative vision to the field.[15] He advocates for normalizing diversity in medicine. He believes that "diversity and inclusion are two different terms. Although Black physicians are hired and represent diversity in a Department, they have to be included as well. It is of utmost importance for them to be part of the conversation for change and to be listened to; they have to be in positions

Table 1
Type of leadership among diverse American Society for Surgery of the Hand and American Association for Hand Surgery presidents

Hand Surgeon	Organization	Period	Type of Leader
Dr Martin A. Entin	ASSH	1973–74	Academic and Society leader, Immigrant
Dr Adrian E. Flatt	ASSH	1975–76	Academic and Society leader, Immigrant
Dr Julio Taleisnik	ASSH	1993–94	Academic and Society leader, Immigrant
Dr Graham Lister	ASSH	1994–95	Academic and Society leader, Immigrant
Dr Marybeth Ezaki	ASSH	2001–02	Academic and Society leader
Dr W.P. Andrew Lee	ASSH AAHS	2011–12 2019–20	Academic, Society, and Innovative leader, Immigrant
Dr Susan E. Mackinnon	AAHS	2005–06	Academic, Society, and Innovative leader
Dr Neil F. Jones	ASSH	2015–16	Academic and Society leader, Immigrant
Dr Ghazi M. Rayan	ASSH	2016–17	Academic, Society leader, Immigrant
Dr James Chang	ASSH	2017–18	Academic, Society, and Innovative leader
Dr Kevin Chung	ASSH	2020–21	Academic, Society and Innovative leader, Immigrant.
Dr Jennifer M. Wolf	ASSH	2022–23	Academic and Society leader

Dr Martin A. Entin was born in the Crimea and immigrated to Canada. Dr Adrian E. Flatt was born in Frinton, England. Dr Julio Taleisnik was born in Argentina. Dr Graham Lister was born in Glasgow, Scotland, with a renowned career. Dr Marybeth Ezaki became the first female president of the ASSH in 2001 and is an expert in congenital hand surgery and brachial plexus birth palsies. Dr Susan E. Mackinnon was the first female president of the AAHS in 2005 and is a peripheral nerve leader and innovator. Dr W.P. Andrew Lee became a leader in hand transplantation and led the surgical team that performed the first double hand transplant and the first above-elbow transplant in the United States. Dr Neil Jones received his medical degree from Oxford University Medical School and trained in general surgery, neurosurgery, and orthopedic surgery in England, becoming a Fellow of the Royal College of Surgeons (FRCS) before his training in the United States. Dr Ghazi Rayan graduated from medical school in Egypt and immigrated to the United States to complete a general surgery internship and orthopedic surgery residency, obtaining prodigious teaching and research experience before becoming president of the ASSH. Dr James Chang, whose parents came from Taiwan, has devoted significant time to advancing the surgical treatment and classification of scleroderma and is currently the Chief of the Division of Plastic and Reconstructive Surgery at Stanford University and became president of ASSH in 2017. Dr Kevin Chung, born in Taiwan, is a true academic leader, developed the Michigan Hand Outcomes Questionnaire, and is also a Society leader. Dr Jennifer Wolf will be the second female ASSH president this upcoming year.

of power to make a difference."[15] He said "in many cases, you need longevity in a Department for this to occur. One needs to obtain tenure."[15]

Types of Leaders

Many categories of leaders have been recognized in the literature; however, in this article we define 3 types of leadership: leadership of position, leadership of innovation, and academic leadership to highlight the great diverse leadership present in Hand Surgery. Noteworthy, many of our giants have practiced one or more of these leadership styles along their professional careers.

Leadership of Position

Leadership positions in Hand Surgery are recognized as presidents of the AAHS and the ASSH, fellowship directors, members of the board and council, journal section editors, and Chairs/Chiefs of Departments, Divisions, or Sections. An overview of our diverse ASSH and AAHS (past and future) presidents has been provided in **Table 1**. As mentioned before, women represent fewer positions in leadership when compared with men (approximately 15% are female); this is fewer than expected based on Hand Surgery fellowship demographic data, in which 25.7% have been female.[10] Gender diversity benefits have been well recognized and include increased sales revenue and innovation.[10] Barriers to diverse leadership include the "glass ceiling phenomenon"; this is where people can rise to a certain level of leadership; however, they cannot seem to break through the highest echelon. Since the foundation of ASSH in 1946, Dr Marybeth Ezaki remains the only female president (served in 2001–02) of this organization until today. Dr Ezaki says that "the society has changed tremendously since then due to the technology in the field of Hand Surgery and medical industrialization in Hand Surgery and believes that the diversity aspect is also gradually changing." It has been recognized by the ASSH that diversity in the field of Hand Surgery is of paramount importance, and efforts have been invested to increase diversity in this field and leadership positions.[16] Dr Ezaki mentions that "you need people to advocate for you and bring you to this next level. If you are doing a good job at your committee, you will likely be asked to move up."

Dr Susan E. Mackinnon, another excellent representative of this category, is the current distinguished Minot Packer Fryer Professor of Plastic Surgery at Washington University School of Medicine in Saint Louis, Missouri. She obtained her medical degree and completed her plastic surgery residency in Canada. Later, she completed her research fellowship in neurologic surgery at the University of Toronto and Hand Surgery fellowship at the Raymond Curtis Hand Center in Baltimore. In 1988, she performed the first nerve allotransplantation using nerves from a cadaver to restore sensation and motor function in a patient with lower extremity nerve injury. Given her well-known expertise in peripheral nerve surgery and her background in basic science research, she has been awarded multiple times and held many leadership positions as President of the American Association of Plastic Surgeons (2008–09), the Plastic Surgery Research Council (1996–97), and the AAHS (2005–06). Despite the difficulties she encountered as a woman in surgery throughout her career, Dr Mackinnon has inspired many women in surgery and has been a strong women's advocate. She said "I hope I have not just broken through the glass ceiling for women, but opened the door and held the door open for them as well." Leadership positions also include being an Editor for Hand Clinics and the Editor-in-Chief of Plastic and Reconstructive Surgery Journal, held by Kevin Chung. He is currently a Professor of Surgery, Plastic Surgery and Orthopedic Surgery at the University of Michigan, Chief of Hand Surgery for Michigan Medicine, and Director of the Comprehensive Hand Center. Not only is he involved in academic leadership but also is actively involved in many other programs such as Global REACH, a global health program that aims to improve health and reduce inequities locally and globally.

Dr Jennifer Wolf, a distinguished orthopedic hand surgeon at the University of Chicago Medical Center, is the next female slated to be president of ASSH from 2022 to 2023. She states that "it is important to diversify Hand Surgery because, similar to other fields, we make better decisions and take better care of patients when we are in an environment that prioritizes diverse backgrounds and points of view." She mentions to her patients and trainees, that residents, fellows and medical students make her better, because "they challenge the thought process, by asking questions, asking why we do things one way and not another." She goes on to say "diversity is just like that; knowing that we are surrounded by others who are distinct and different from us, pushes us to consider other solutions or views and allows us to broaden our worldview and knowledge. This is key to growth and evolution in Hand Surgery." We hope that the number of diverse leaders increases over the next few years to better represent the demographics of hand surgeons and the patients they serve.

Dr Ghazi Rayan's main theme of his ASSH presidency (2016–17) was diversity. He mentioned to be "living proof that the organization of ASSH is a melting pot. It rewards assiduous work, opens doors of opportunities to anyone regardless of their background." To this end, he has recently written a book titled "Immigrants Who Founded and Fostered an Early Nation."

Leadership of Innovation

Historically, the field of surgery has taken significant pride in leading the profession in safety, quality, innovation, and education. Surgical innovation is defined as "the development of a new procedure or technology used for a procedure, the development of a substantial modification of an existing procedure or technology, or the application of an existing procedure, technology or product for a new indication."[17] These advances would only be expected to lead the way for enhancement of racial and ethnic diversity in our field.[18] Dr W.P. Andrew Lee, Dean of the University of Texas Southwestern Medical School and executive vice president for academic affairs and provost of UT Southwestern Medical Center, grew up in Taiwan before coming to the United States at age 15 years. He quickly assimilated and excelled, attending Harvard College before medical school and residency at Johns Hopkins University. He led teams that completed the nation's first double hand transplant, first above-elbow transplant, and the world's first total penis and scrotum transplant. Moreover, Dr Lee has served in leadership positions of the ASSH, American Board of Plastic Surgery, the American Society for Reconstructive Transplantation, and the AAHS. We recognize Dr Lee as one of our innovative leaders in the field of Hand Surgery. Dr James Chang is currently the Johnson & Johnson Distinguished Professor and Chief of the Division of Plastic and Reconstructive Surgery at Stanford University. Dr Chang may be recognized for his presidential leadership of the ASSH (2017–18), his academic accomplishments, and his efforts in community work (Resurge International) among his many achievements. As an innovator, he and his team recently established a new scleroderma classification system based on angiograms of the hand in patients with systemic sclerosis.[19] He mentions that "a good leader creates a team with the best people in each field and lets smart people do what they do. The leader's job is to remove the barriers, share the work and share the credit."

Similarly, we honor Dr Jorge L. Orbay as one of our innovative leaders. Dr Orbay graduated from the University of Puerto Rico, received his residency training at the Hospital for Joint Diseases Orthopedic Institute of New York, and completed his fellowship in hand and microsurgery at the University of Miami Jackson Memorial Hospital. He is currently the medical director at Miami Hand & Upper Extremity Institute located in Miami and is well-recognized for introducing the concept of volar fixed-angle plating for the treatment of distal radius fractures. Other examples include but are not limited to Dr Luis R. Scheker and Dr Lisa Lattanza. Dr Scheker graduated from the University of Santo Domingo and completed his postgraduate training in London, Scotland, and the United States. He is currently an Associate Professor of Surgery at the University of Louisville and Assistant Consulting Professor of surgery at Duke University, and well known for developing artificial joints to replace the distal radioulnar joint, radio ulnar/radio carpal joint, and the proximal radio ulnar joint of the forearm.[20] Dr Lisa Lattanza, Chair of the Department of Orthopedics and Rehabilitation at the Yale School of Medicine and an active leader in Hand Surgery, has been a leader in 3D surgical planning and technology for deformity correction and led the team that performed the first elbow-to-elbow transplant in the world.[21] Dr Lattanza was also actively involved in teaching, promoting the involvement of women in the field in the early stages of their life. We believe that innovation is a powerful tool to become a leader in the field. However, this does not follow a linear pattern. Dr Mackinnon, who is also an innovator of Nerve Surgery, delineated that innovation is not always welcome. She said "when you innovate, there will be people from the previous paradigm, wanting to support a push back." Although this may happen, the ability to innovate moves the field forward and provides better care to our patients.

Academic Leadership

Academic leadership is defined as the commitment to teaching, learning, research productivity, and academic performance.[22] Research productivity is usually linked to this definition as this leader creates ideas, sets a vision, and inspires people to invest in research.[23] Lately, with efforts to increase diversity, research and time are becoming crucial for underrepresented physicians to be able to reach equal representation at the highest positions of an organization.[24] Most of our diverse Hand Surgery giants actively participate in this type of leadership. Many leaders lean toward the academic field given the fact that they find it enjoyable to teach, mentor, advise, and train medical students and residents who will become our future leaders. The academic environment allows for influencing society by training good surgeons, as Dr Armstrong supports.[15]

Dr Augusta Déjerine-Klumpke (1859–1927) may have been the first great example of this type of leadership. The name Klumpke is well known throughout the medical field, denoting Klumpke palsy or lower trunk brachial plexopathy.[25] Despite familiarity with the injury, many physicians are unfamiliar with the woman who described this condition. Her achievements take on added significance because of the difficulties to enter the medical field as a woman at that time. She is seen as pioneer in the history of French feminism and was the first women selected as an intern in the Paris hospitals. While reviewing her legacy, we recognize the obstacles that she had to overcome to enter academic medicine. Augusta was supported by Professor Vulpian (a French neurologist and codiscoverer of spinal muscular atrophy). She received her doctoral degree, was awarded numerous prizes, and helped standardize protocols for the care of paraplegic patients. As a pioneer in the rehabilitation of spinal cord injury, she overcame all challenges that came to her, not only as a women of her era but also as a scientist and physician of the highest caliber.[26] Nearly a century after Klumpke's death, we are still facing many of the same challenges for women in leadership positions.

The academic environment still faces many challenges related to microaggressions due to race and gender; however, it is gradually changing. Dr Mackinnon shared with us that the most challenging thing for her was "having a sense of not fully belonging as a woman in a man's game." Despite these challenges, efforts have been invested in promoting equity and inclusion in the academic fields.

How to Improve Diversity in Hand Surgery

When looking at the impact that one can make, we must start small. Making changes on the department level will eventually lead to changes in the field. It is suggested by Dr Kerri Woodberry, hand surgeon and Chief of Plastic Surgery at

West Virginia University, that when recruiting diverse faculty and trainees, institutions need to implement implicit bias training for faculty members and truly look at applicants' qualities and characteristics, and not just at metrics.[27] Diversity drives excellence by inherently incorporating diverse thoughts, backgrounds, and perspectives. It has been demonstrated that diversity improves the patient-physician relationship, cross-cultural communication, and patient satisfaction.[28,29] On the other hand, lack of diversity has a negative effect on patient care, the culture of our health care system, and research productivity.[11] To create that change, "we need to be proactive and intentional with our diversity efforts" as stated by our senior author, Dr Moore. We can only benefit from diversity by leaning in and committing to it. This means avoiding all male or all White panels, webinars, and speakers. We have to think broader and include new faces. When nomination slates are not reflective of the organization or lack diversity, we have to push back. We need to move past the "known and give" others a chance. These wise words reflect the accepting culture in the department that Dr Moore leads.

Fostering diversity in our field is essential for continued excellence. We may need to rethink how we select the next generation of Hand surgeons to achieve diversity. Dr Lisa Lattanza said "We have studied what correlates most highly with becoming a successful surgeon and added those skills and attributes to the selection criteria for residents. For example, grit and resilience correlate more highly with success as a surgeon than board scores. Research supports the characteristics and life experiences that score highly on the grit/resilience scale. We are not just saying, you get more points because you're a woman or a minority," she said. "We're weighting things toward people who have a more interesting story, a different path and this leads to a more diverse residency class."[30] Excellence and the desire to achieve your goals are personal and come from an internal drive to be the best version of yourself that you can be, every day. This is independent of race, gender, sexual orientation, or religious preference.

"As a profession, we have invested a significant amount of money and time into pipeline programs and those are all wonderful endeavors," as mentioned by Dr Erica Taylor, Assistant Professor of Orthopedic Hand and Upper Extremity Surgery at Duke University. The impact of these efforts often takes several years to be observed and measured. What needs to happen in the "now" is a critical examination and renovation of the systemic processes and practices that we have in place throughout our organizations. How do we search and select talent? How is our leadership held accountable for owning this space and being part of the change? How is pay equity evaluated and then repaired? These questions and many more remain to be answered in the upcoming years in our search to improve and diversify our field. The opportunities for systematic change are endless; however, we have not emphasized the leadership skills required to change organizational culture in health care. In 2020, Dr Taylor founded the Orthopedic Diversity Leadership Consortium (ODLC) to empower clinical leaders of diversity to recognize and understand these structural opportunities and implement sustainable strategic change. Lenses of equity and inclusion need to be embedded in all strategic decisions that are being made in our health care facilities and organizations. We believe that these efforts will eventually benefit our colleagues, our leaders, and above all, our patients.

SUMMARY

Diverse leadership exists in Hand Surgery; however, we recognize not only the uphill battle but also the diverse perspectives of those who have broken through barriers. Strong efforts are being invested into diversifying Hand Surgery because diversity drives excellence by inherently incorporating diverse thoughts, backgrounds, and perspectives. We are confident that with these efforts, the number of diverse leaders will continue to increase, and success will be redefined.

ACKNOWLEDGMENTS

The authors thank our leaders for sharing their stories. Approval of this article has been provided by all featured leaders.

DISCLOSURE

None.

REFERENCES

1. Van Vugt M. Evolutionary origins of leadership and followership. Pers Soc Psychol Rev 2006;10(4):354–71.
2. Bass BM. The leaderless group discussion. Psychol Bull 1954;51(5):465–92.
3. Hollander EP, Julian JW. Contemporary trends in the analysis of leadership processes. Psychol Bull 1969;71(5):387–97.
4. Goleman D, Boyatzis R, McKee A. Primal leadership: The hidden driver of great performance. Harv

Business Rev 2001;. https://hbr.org/2001/12/primal-leadership-the-hidden-driver-of-great-performance.

5. Kassam AF, Taylor M, Cortez AR, et al. Gender and ethnic diversity in academic general surgery department leadership. Am J Surg 2021;221(2):363–8.
6. Morris-Wiseman LF, Cañez C, Romero Arenas MA, et al. Race, Gender, and International Medical Graduates: Leadership Trends in Academic Surgical Societies. J Surg Res 2022;270:430–6.
7. Poon S, Abzug J, Caird M, et al. A Five-year Review of the Designated Leadership Positions of Pediatric Orthopaedic Society of North America: Where Do Women Stand? Orthop Clin North Am 2019;50(3):331–5.
8. Emamaullee JA, Lyons MV, Berdan E, et al. Women leaders in surgery: past, present, and future. Bull Am Coll Surg 2012;97(8):24–9.
9. Carr PL, Gunn CM, Kaplan SA, et al. Inadequate progress for women in academic medicine: findings from the National Faculty Study. J Womens Health (Larchmt) 2015;24(3):190–9.
10. Brisbin AK, Chen W, Goldschmidt E, et al. Gender Diversity in Hand Surgery Leadership. Hand (N Y) 2022. https://doi.org/10.1177/15589447211038679. 15589447211038679.
11. Bae GH, Lee AW, Park DJ, et al. Ethnic and gender diversity in hand surgery trainees. J Hand Surg Am 2015;40(4):790–7.
12. Duckworth A. Grit: the power of passion and perseverance. New York: Scribner; 2016.
13. Triandis HC. The future of workforce diversity in international organisations: A commentary. Appl Psychol 2003;52(3):486–95.
14. Mayer RC, Warr RS, Zhao J. Do Pro-Diversity Policies Improve Corporate Innovation? Financial Management 2017;47(3):617–50.
15. Showly Nicholson DB. Surgeon Spotlight: Dr. Milton Armstrong. https://garnessociety.org/surgeon-spotlight-1-dr-milton-armstrong/. Accessed 4 June 2022.
16. Earp BE, Mora AN, Rozental TD. Extending a Hand: Increasing Diversity at the American Society for Surgery of the Hand. J Hand Surg Am 2018;43(7):649–56.
17. Dengler J, Padovano WM, Davidge K, et al. Dissemination and Implementation Science in Plastic and Reconstructive Surgery: Perfecting, Protecting, and Promoting the Innovation That Defines Our Specialty. Plast Reconstr Surg 2021;147(2):303e–13e.
18. Butler PD, Aarons CB, Ahn J, et al. Leading From the Front: An Approach to Increasing Racial and Ethnic Diversity in Surgical Training Programs. Ann Surg 2019;269(6):1012–5.
19. Leyden J, Burn MB, Wong V, et al. Upper Extremity Angiographic Patterns in Systemic Sclerosis: Implications for Surgical Treatment. J Hand Surg 2019; 44(11):990.e991–7.
20. Luis R. Scheker, MD. Available at: https://christinemkleinertinstitute.org/about/faculty/luis-r-scheker-md/. Accessed June 4, 2022.
21. Lisa Lattanza, MD, FAOA, FAAOS. Available at: https://medicine.yale.edu/profile/lisa_lattanza/. Accessed June 4, 2022.
22. Saroyan A, Getahun D, Gebre E. Understanding academic leadership. 2011. Available at: https://www.researchgate.net/publication/269947011.
23. Ball S. Leadership of Academics in Research. Educ Management Adm Leadersh 2007;35(4):449–77.
24. McCullough M, Willacy RA, Luong M, et al. A 5-Year Review of the Designated Leadership Positions of the American Society for Surgery of the Hand (ASSH). J Hand Surg Am 2021;46(2):151.e1-5.
25. Merryman J, Varacallo M. Klumpke palsy. Treasure Island (FL): StatPearls; 2022.
26. Ulgen BO, Brumblay H, Yang LJ, et al. Augusta Dejerine-Klumpke, M.D. (1859-1927): a historical perspective on Klumpke's palsy. Neurosurgery 2008;63(2):359–66 [discussion: 366–7].
27. Lane J. Mentor Spotlight: Dr. Kerri woodberry. Available at: https://www.womensurgeons.org/news/561714/Mentor-Spotlight-Dr.-Kerri-Woodberry.htm#:~:text=Kerri%20Woodberry%20is%20an%20associate,plastic%20surgery%2C%20and%20hand%20surgery. Accessed June 4, 2022.
28. Cooper-Patrick L, Gallo JJ, Gonzales JJ, et al. Race, gender, and partnership in the patient-physician relationship. Jama 1999;282(6):583–9.
29. Menendez ME, Loeffler M, Ring D. Patient Satisfaction in an Outpatient Hand Surgery Office: A Comparison of English- and Spanish-Speaking Patients. Qual Manag Health Care 2015;24(4):183–9.
30. McFarling UL. Orthopedic surgeons pride themselves on fixing things. Can they fix their own field's lack of diversity?. Available at: https://www.statnews.com/2021/12/14/orthopedic-surgeons-fixing-their-fields-lack-of-diversity/. Accessed June 4, 2022.

The Value of Diversity, Equity, and Inclusion
Race and Ethnicity Affecting Patients

Christopher O. Bayne, MD

KEYWORDS

• Diversity • Race • Ethnicity • Hand Surgery • Patients • Outcomes

KEY POINTS

- The Unites States is becoming increasingly diverse.
- Although diversity in Medicine and Hand Surgery is increasing, it is not matching the diversity of the population as a whole.
- Patient race and ethnicity are important factors in health-care inequity in the United States.
- Physician diversity is associated with improved patient care.
- Increasing and maintaining physician diversity in Hand surgery is paramount.

BACKGROUND

Since 2010, the racial and ethnic diversity of the United States has increased significantly, with the results of the 2020 US Census revealing that diversity is increasing in 19 of every 20 US counties.[1,2] This trend is projected to continue, with the overall White population decreasing for the first time in history and most people aged younger than 18 years identifying as other than White (including multiracial, Hispanic, Asian, or Black).[1] As of 2020, non-Latino White people make up 57.8% of the United States population compared with 63% in 2010.[3,4]

Traditionally, the diversity of the United States populace has not been mirrored by the demographics of the physicians who care for it. For example, in 2018, although those identifying as Black numbered about 13% of the population, only 5% of physicians identified as Black.[5] Although those identifying as Hispanic or Latino numbered about 18% population, only 5.8% of physicians identified as Hispanic or Latino.[5] Only 0.3% of physicians identified as American Indian or Alaskan native and 0.1% as Hawaiian native or Pacific Islander.[5]

Data on the demographics of practicing Hand surgeons are less available but a recent American Association for Surgery of the Hand abstract presenting the results of a study calculating the racial and ethnic diversity among faculty Hand Surgeons and fellows at academic centers reported that 75.6% were White.[6] This suggests that Hand Surgeons practicing in the United States are significantly less diverse than the country as a whole.

To understand the value of diversity in Hand surgery, it is important to recognize how the race and ethnicity of both patients and physicians affect the delivery of care.

PATIENT RACE AND ETHNICITY

According to the American Psychological Association, the term race refers to physical differences that groups and cultures consider socially significant, whereas the term ethnicity refers to shared cultural characteristics including language, ancestry, practices, and beliefs.[7]

Patient race and ethnicity are important factors in health-care inequity in the United States, with significant demographic disparities in coverage, chronic health conditions, and mortality.[8] For example, African American men have the lowest life expectancy of any group in the United States,[9] living less than non-Hispanic White men by an average of 4.5 years.[10,11]

Department of Orthopaedic Surgery, University of California, Davis, 4860 Y Street, Suite 3800, Sacramento, CA 95817, USA
E-mail address: cbayne@ucdavis.edu

Hand Clin 39 (2023) 9–15
https://doi.org/10.1016/j.hcl.2022.08.001

Differences in poverty level and access to resources exist across racial and ethnic groups[12] but differences in morbidity, mortality, quality of life, and disability exist despite controlling for socioeconomic status.[13–17] The reasons for these disparities are complex and multifactorial, including long-standing systematic inequalities in housing, economics, and health-care systems.[8,11,18,19] In Hand surgery, we frequently witness these complex factors affect patient care (**Figs. 1** and **2**). It can be helpful to consider the effects of race and ethnicity on patient care in Hand surgery and in general by examining differences in access, quality of care, and outcomes.[20]

ACCESS TO CARE

Disparities in access to care have been well documented in the Orthopedic Surgery and Plastic Surgery literature. Skolasky and colleagues reported a lower rate of hospitalization for lumbar spinal stenosis surgery for Black and Hispanic patients compared with White patients,[21] and Zhang and coinvestigators found significantly lower total knee arthroplasty rates among non-White patients as well as a lower likelihood of non-White patients to have arthroplasty surgery at a high volume hospital.[22] Butler and colleagues found that women of color who lived in regions of high plastic surgeon density and had private insurance had postmastectomy breast reconstruction rates that were 25% lower than Caucasian women living in similar circumstances.[23]

Although there are fewer published studies, existing evidence demonstrate that the same disparities exist in hand and upper extremity surgery. Eichinger reported a 54% lower utilization rate for shoulder arthroplasty among Black patients and a 74% lower utilization rate among Hispanic patients compared with White patients.[24] Brodeur and colleagues found that Non-White and Hispanic patients with carpal tunnel syndrome had lower odds of carpal tunnel release than White, non-Hispanic patients.[25] The authors reported similar findings in the management of trigger finger in their abstract presented at a recent American Association for Hand Surgery annual meeting, with non-White patients having lower odds of surgical release than White patients.[26]

In order to improve access to care, it is first important that Hand Surgeons understand that disparities in access exist. Second, it is important that they recognize that they are not uncommon. Although some differences in access may be attributable to geographic differences, the literature demonstrates that there are disparities across racial and ethnic groups for patients treated within the same medical center, at major medical centers, and across socio-economic lines.[22–26] As such, it may be beneficial for the Hand surgeon to reflect on how differences in access to care can affect patients within his or her own practice. Although systemic inequities are likely to contribute significantly,[8,11,18,19] it is only when we evaluate our own practices that we will be able to address barriers to care at the individual level.

QUALITY OF CARE

Commonly cited measures of quality include, but are not limited to, experience of care, preventive care, chronic disease control, and hospitalizations.[27] It is well documented that quality of care is influenced by race and ethnicity.[27–34]

The National Consumer Assessment of Health Plans (CAHPS) data demonstrate that Asian Americans, especially those with limited English proficiency, report lower experience of care rates compared with White patients.[27–29] An analysis of Medicare data revealed that Black beneficiaries

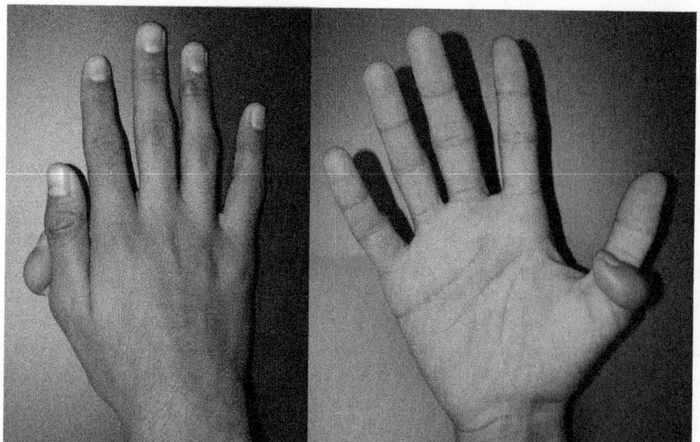

Fig. 1. A 16-year-old Latino boy who presented with a right thumb preaxial polydactyly. This resulted in significant pain over the years and was removed via WALANT approach in clinic with immediate relief of pain and discomfort. The child kept this extra digit without initially seeking surgical care because of cultural issues and the fear of general anesthesia. (*Courtesy of Michael Galvez, MD, Madera, CA*)

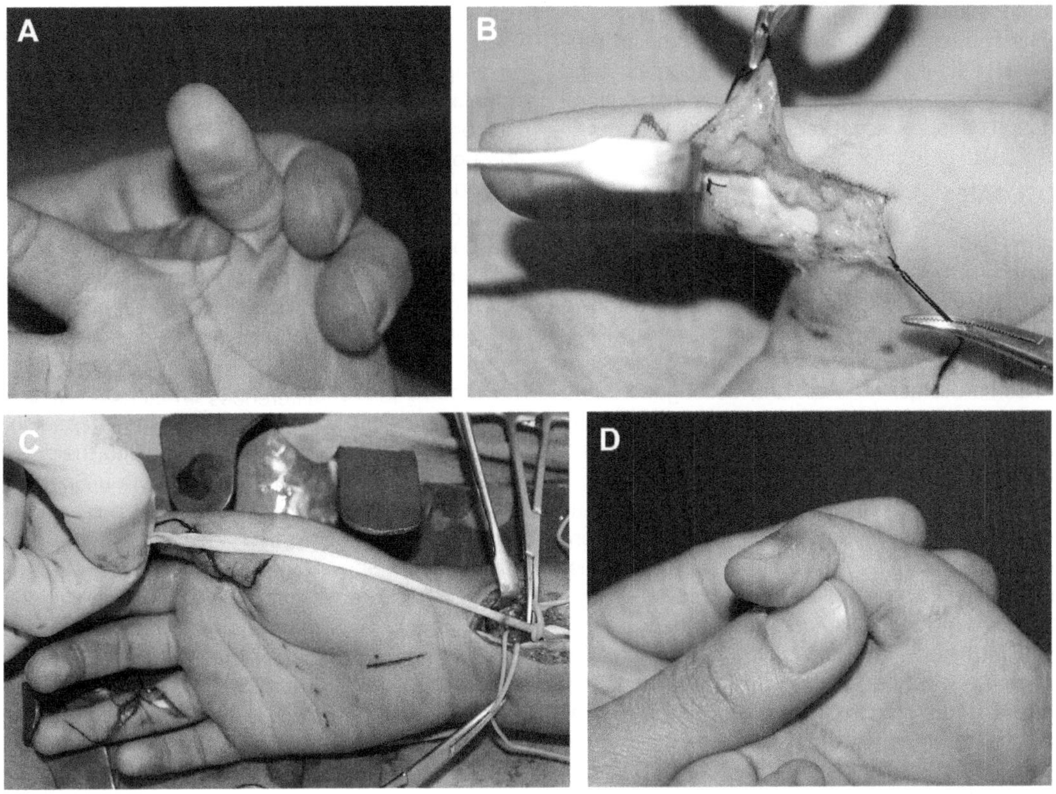

Fig. 2. A 5-year-old Latina girl who presented 2 years after sharp laceration of her right thumb and presented with inability to flex her dominant right thumb at the interphalangeal joint (*A*). She underwent staged flexor tendon reconstruction with hunter rod placement (*B*). Given a fibrosed flexor pollicis longus tendon she underwent second stage reconstruction with ring finger flexor digitorum profundus tendon transfer (*C*). Her postoperative recovery was complicated by missed appointments but ultimately, she did develop full and complete function of her right thumb interphalangeal joint with active flexion (*D*). This child had delayed care secondary to socioeconomic challenges, complex social situation, and difficulty with traveling resulting in delayed care. (*Courtesy of Michael Galvez, MD, Madera, CA*)

received only 4 nonelective procedures more frequently than White beneficiaries (lower limb amputation, debridement, arteriovenostomy, and bilateral testicle removal)—all of which were suggestive of higher rates of delayed diagnosis or failure in management of chronic disease.[30,31]

Similar findings are present in the Hand Surgery literature. In their analysis of CAHPS data, Menendez and colleagues found that compared with primarily English-speaking patients, primarily Spanish-speaking patients were less likely to be satisfied with the care provided in a Hand Surgery office.[32] This included lower satisfaction with provider listening and with provider spending enough time during visits.[32] Attempt at replantation surgery is less likely for Black and Hispanic children than for White children, despite controlling for confounding factors.[33] Mahmoudi and colleagues demonstrated similar findings in adult patients, with African American patients being less likely to undergo replantation procedures than White patients despite controlling for patient and hospital characteristics.[34]

In their analysis on racial and ethnic disparities in health-care quality, Fiscella and Sanders document that health-care disparities are a result of the combination of social disadvantage and insufficient health-care system responsiveness to this disadvantage.[27] Although eliminating these disparities will require commitment at a national level, local quality improvement strategies that engage patients, communities, and clinicians can have a positive impact.[27] This can include efforts to ensure excellent communication with patients. For example, Hand Surgery practices can work to guarantee the availability of translating services for their patients who do not speak English. In addition, patients who speak a language that is different from that of their provider may require more time during visits to confirm appropriate understanding and patient satisfaction. It is important that health-care interventions are explained well for all patient populations, and Hand Surgeons should ensure that the discussion of procedure details, expectations, outcomes, and complications consider potential patient cultural differences in the acceptability of these factors.

OUTCOMES

Many studies across specialties suggest disparities in health-care outcomes based on race and ethnicity.[22,35–42] Willer and colleagues have shown that Black and Hispanic children are more likely than White children to die after surgery regardless of income status.[35,36] Azin and colleagues found increased morbidity, mortality, and readmissions for Black patients across surgical specialties and procedures.[37]

Although there are few Hand Surgery publications that directly examine the effect of patient race and ethnicity on outcomes, the data that exist suggest similar disparities.[38] Jawad and colleagues found worse outcome for non-White patients with bone sarcoma of the hand and wrist compared with White patients.[38] Contrastingly, the orthopedic surgery, plastic surgery, and general surgery literature is notable for numerous studies that demonstrate outcome disparities.[22,39–42] Because Hand Surgery is a subspecialty of orthopedic, plastic, and general surgery, it is logical that additional Hand Surgery studies would have comparable findings.

Although there is potential for inherent systemic issues such as health-care provider and health-care system biases to influence a patient's disposition and outcome,[37] the Hand surgeon who is aware of this potential for outcome disparities may be inspired to examine the diversity within his or her own patient population. This may allow Hand Surgeons to address possible causes of outcome differences within their own practices. For example, as Azin and colleagues underscore, Black patients may be less likely to have access to meaningful community supports that facilitate remaining at home after discharge.[37] Minority patients may benefit from more longitudinal and multidisciplinary disposition planning including social work, discharge coordinators, and nurse navigators.[43]

PHYSICIAN DIVERSITY

Although patient race and ethnicity have been shown to be correlated with poor access, quality, and outcomes, the benefits of physician racial and ethnic diversity have been well documented in the medical literature.[44–50] Physician diversity has been shown to promote better access to care and improve health-care quality and satisfaction for underserved populations.[44,45] For example, Black and Hispanic physicians are significantly more likely to practice in underserved minority communities than physicians from other groups.[46] Concordance, most often defined as a similarity or shared identity between physician and patient based on a demographic attribute, has been shown to have a positive influence on disparities in medical care, improving usage, communication, and patient satisfaction.[47] Minority patients with physicians of similar ethnicity are more likely to rate their physicians as excellent, to receive preventative care, and to be satisfied with their health care overall.[48] Spanish-speaking patients report greater satisfaction with their care when they communicate directly with a Spanish-speaking physician than through professional interpreter services with a non–Spanish-speaking physician.[49] Some studies also suggest improvement in health-care outcomes for minority patients with patient–physician race concordance but this data are mixed and inconclusive.[51]

Compared with primary care, fewer studies evaluate the effect of patient–physician racial and ethnic concordance in the subspecialty setting. In one of the few published studies, Kamal and colleagues found that patients value concordance in subspecialty care as much as they do in primary care.[50] Although it did not specifically evaluate patient–physician concordance in hand and upper extremity surgery, the study was conducted at a multispecialty Orthopedic Surgery clinic that included Hand Surgery care.[50]

It is clear that is if we are to improve patient care for all populations, we must make physician diversity a priority.

SUMMARY

As Hand Surgeons, it is our goal to provide the best care for our patients. If we are to do so, it is imperative that we work to ensure and maintain diversity within our specialty. Fortunately, strides are being made in this regard. The class of students entering medical school in 2021 was more diverse than any historically preceding class.[52] In addition, in a study analyzing graduate medical education demographic data between 1995 and 2012, Bae and colleagues found that diversity has increased significantly in Hand Surgery trainees.[3] However, more action is necessary. Wo and colleagues' study revealing the current lack of diversity among Hand Surgeons and Hand Surgery fellows[6] demonstrates that much work remains if we are make our field as diverse as the patients that we care for. This may be facilitated through measures such as making diversity a goal across our institutions.[3,53] (As an example the American Society for Surgery of the Hand has a Diversity and Inclusion statement, a Diversity Task Force, and gives a platform for educational topics on Diversity, Equity, and Inclusion at the Annual Conference.) Additional measures, such as increasing exposure of students at the undergraduate and medical school level to Hand Surgery, bringing attention to the work and careers of minority Hand Surgeons and trainees, and highlighting opportunities in Hand Surgery to care for underserved populations may attract more minority applicants.[54] It is also important that we ensure that those people of color that do decide to pursue a career in Hand Surgery know that they belong, are wanted in our specialty, and are able to train and practice in a supportive environment.[54]

These efforts are necessary if we are to provide the excellent care that our patients deserve to *all* of our patient populations.

DISCLOSURE

Dr C.O. Bayne or an immediate family member serves as a paid consultant to LimaCorporate. Dr C.O. Bayne has not received anything of value from or has stock or stock options held in a commercial company or institution related directly or indirectly to the subject of this article.

REFERENCES

1. Bureau USC. 2020 U . S . Population More Racially and Ethnically Diverse Than Measured in 2010. 2021. Available at: https://www.census.gov/library/stories/2021/08/2020-united-states-population-more-racially-ethnically-diverse-than-2010.html.
2. Tavernise S, Gebeloff R. Census Shows sharply Growing Numbers of Hispanic, Asian and multiracial Americans. New York Times; 2021. Available at: https://www.nytimes.com/2021/08/12/us/us-census-population-growth-diversity.html.
3. Bae GH, Lee AW, Park DJ, et al. Ethnic and gender diversity in hand surgery trainees. J Hand Surg Am 2015;40(4):790–7.
4. United States Census Bureau. Racial and Ethnic Diversity in the United States: 2010 Census and 2020 Census. 2021;(X):2020-2021. Available at: https://www.census.gov/library/visualizations/interactive/racial-and-ethnic-diversity-in-the-united-states-2010-and-2020-census.html.
5. AAMC. Diversity in Medicine: Facts and Figures 2019. Assoc Am Med Coll 2019;20001. Available at: https://www.aamc.org/data-reports/workforce/interactive-data/figure-18-percentage-all-active-physicians-race/ethnicity-2018.
6. Wo LM, Smith KL, Plana NM, et al. Current Diversity in Academic Hand Surgery. Koloa, HI: Am Assoc hand Surg Annu Meet; 2021.
7. American Psychological Association. Racial and Ethnic Identity. 2022. Available at: https://apastyle.apa.org/style-grammar-guidelines/bias-free-language/racial-ethnic-minorities.
8. Carratala S, Maxwell C. Health Disparities by Race and Ethnicity. Cent Am Prog 2020;1–8. October 2018.
9. Arias E, Heron M, Xu J. United States Life Tables, 2013. Natl Vital Stat Rep 2017;66(3):1–64.
10. Murphy SL, Xu J, Kochanek KD, et al. Deaths: Final data for 2015. Natl Vital Stat Rep 2017;66(6). https://doi.org/10.1136/vr.h753.
11. Alsan M, Garrick O, Graziani G. Does diversity matter for health? Experimental evidence from Oakland. Am Econ Rev 2019;109(12):4071–111.
12. Creamer J. Poverty Rates for Blacks and Hispanics Reached Historic Lows in 2019. US Census Bur 2020. Available at: https://www.census.gov/library/stories/2020/09/poverty-rates-for-blacks-and-hispanics-reached-historic-lows-in-2019.html.
13. Ferraro KF, Farmer MM. Double Jeopardy to Health Hypothesis for African Americans: Analysis and Critique. J Health Soc Behav 1996;37(1):27–43.
14. Winkleby MA, Kraemer HC, Ahn DK, et al. Ethnic and socioeconomic differences in cardiovascular disease risk factors: Findings for women from the third national health and nutrition examination survey, 1988-1994. J Am Med Assoc 1998;280(4):356–62.
15. Clark DO, Maddox GL. Racial and Social Correlates of Age-Related Changes in Functioning. J Gentrology 1992;47(5):S222–32.
16. Hughes M, Thomas ME. The continuing significance of race revisited: A study of race, class, and quality of life in America, 1972 to 1996. Am Sociol Rev 1998;63(6):785–95.
17. Farmer MM, Ferraro KF. Are racial disparities in health conditional on socioeconomic status? Soc Sci Med 2005;60(1):191–204.
18. Smedley BD, Stith AY, Nelson AR. Unequal Treatment: Confronting Racial and Ethnic Disparities in Health Care (with CD). Unequal Treat Confronting Racial Ethn Disparities Heal Care (With Cd) 2003;(Cdc):1–764.
19. Malizos KN, Dailiana ZH, Innocenti M, et al. Vascularized bone grafts for upper limb reconstruction: Defects at the distal radius, wrist, and hand. J Hand Surg Am 2010;35(10):1710–8.
20. Pandya NK, Wustrack R, Metz L, et al. Current concepts in orthopaedic care disparities. J Am Acad Orthop Surg 2018;26(23):823–32.
21. Skolasky RL, Maggard AM, Thorpe RJ, et al. United States hospital admissions for lumbar spinal stenosis: Racial and ethnic differences, 2000 through 2009. Spine (Phila Pa 1976) 2013;38(26):2272–8.

22. Zhang W, Lyman S, Boutin-Foster C, et al. Racial and ethnic disparities in utilization rate, hospital volume, and perioperative outcomes after total knee arthroplasty. J Bone Jt Surg - Am 2016;98(15):1243–52.
23. Butler PD, Familusi O, Serletti JM, et al. Influence of race, insurance status, and geographic access to plastic surgeons on immediate breast reconstruction rates. Am J Surg 2018;215(6):987–94.
24. Eichinger JK, Greenhouse AR, Rao MV, et al. Racial and sex disparities in utilization rates for shoulder arthroplasty in the United States disparities in shoulder arthroplasty. J Orthop 2019;16(3):195–200.
25. Brodeur PG, Patel DD, Licht AH, et al. Demographic Disparities amongst Patients Receiving Carpal Tunnel Release: A Retrospective Review of 92,921 Patients. Plast Reconstr Surg - Glob Open 2021; 9(11):E3959.
26. Brodeur PG, Patel DD, Raducha JE, et al. Social disparities in the management of trigger finger: an analysis of 31,411 Cases. Carlsbad, (CA): Am Assoc Hand Surg Annu Meetting; 2022.
27. Fiscella K, Sanders MR. Racial and Ethnic Disparities in the Quality of Health Care. Annu Rev Public Health 2016;37:375–94.
28. Goldstein E, Elliott MN, Lehrman WG, et al. Racial/ethnic differences in patients' perceptions of inpatient care using the HCAHPS survey. Med Care Res Rev 2010;67(1):74–92.
29. Morales LS, Elliott MN, Weech-Maldonado R, et al. Differences in CAHPS adult survey reports and ratings by race and ethnicity: an analysis of the National CAHPS benchmarking data 1.0. Health Serv Res 2001;36(3):595–617. http://www.ncbi.nlm.nih.gov/pubmed/11482591%0Ahttp://www.pubmedcentral.nih.gov/articlerender.fcgi?artid=PMC1089244.
30. McBean AM, Gornick M. Differences by race in the rates of procedures performed in hospitals for Medicare beneficiaries. Health Care Financ Rev 1994; 15(4):77–90.
31. National Research Council. In: Bulatao RA, Anderson NB, editors. Understanding racial and ethnic differences in health in late life: a Research Agenda. Washington, DC: The National Academies Press; 2004.
32. Menendez ME, Loeffler M, Ring D. Patient satisfaction in an outpatient hand surgery office: A comparison of english- and Spanish-speaking patients. Qual Manag Health Care 2015;24(4):183–9.
33. Lee S, Reichert H, Kim HM, et al. Patterns of surgical care and health disparities of treating pediatric finger amputation injuries in the United States. J Am Coll Surg 2011;213(4):475–85.
34. Mahmoudi E, Swiatek PR, Chung KC, et al. Racial Variation in Treatment of Traumatic Finger/Thumb Amputation: A National Comparative Study of Replantation and Revision Amputation. Plast Reconstr Surg 2016;137(3):576e–85e.
35. Willer BL, Mpody C, Tobias JD, et al. Association of Race and Family Socioeconomic Status With Pediatric Postoperative Mortality. JAMA Netw Open 2022; 5(3):e222989.
36. Willer BL, Mpody C, Tobias JD, et al. Racial Disparities in Pediatric Surgical Mortality Accross the Spectrum of Socioeconomic Status. New Orleans, LA: Anesthesiol Annu Meet; 2021.
37. Azin A, Hirpara DH, Doshi S, et al. Racial Disparities in Surgery. Ann Surg Open 2020;1(2):e023.
38. Jawad MU, Bayne CO, Farhan S, et al. Prognostic factors, disparity, and equity variables impacting prognosis in bone sarcomas of the hand: SEER database review. J Surg Oncol 2021;124(8): 1515–22.
39. Schoenfeld AJ, Zhang D, Walley KC, et al. The influence of race and hospital environment on the care of patients with cervical spine fractures. Spine J 2016; 16(5):602–7.
40. Hauc SC, Junn A, Dinis J, et al. Disparities in Craniosynostosis Outcomes by Race and Insurance Status. J Craniofac Surg 2022;33(1):121–4.
41. Peck CJ, Pourtaheri N, Shultz BN, et al. Racial Disparities in Complications, Length of Stay, and Costs Among Patients Receiving Orthognathic Surgery in the United States. J Oral Maxillofac Surg 2021; 79(2):441–9.
42. Falcone M, Liu L, Farias A, et al. Evidence for racial/ethnic disparities in emergency department visits following breast cancer surgery among women in California: a population-based study. Breast Cancer Res Treat 2021;187(3):831–41.
43. Ko N, Snyder F, Raich P, et al. Racial and Ethnic Differences in Patient Navigation: Results from the Patient Navigation Research Program. Cancer 2016; 122(17):2715–22.
44. Marrast LM, Zallman L, Woolhandler S, et al. Minority physicians' role in the care of underserved patients: Diversifying the physicianworkforce may be key in addressing health disparities. JAMA Intern Med 2014;174(2):289–91.
45. Takeshita J, Wang S, Loren AW, et al. Association of Racial/Ethnic and Gender Concordance Between Patients and Physicians With Patient Experience Ratings. JAMA Netw Open 2020;3(11):e2024583.
46. Komaromy M, Grumbach K, Drake M, et al. The Role of Black and Hispanic Physicians in Providing Health Care for Underserved Populations. N Engl J Med 1996;334(20):1305–10.
47. Street RL, O'Malley KJ, Cooper LA, et al. Understanding concordance in patient-physician relationships: Personal and ethnic dimensions of shared identity. Ann Fam Med 2008;6(3):198–205.
48. Saha S, Komaromy M, Koepsell TD, et al. Patient-physician racial concordance and the perceived quality and use of health care. Arch Intern Med 1999;159(9):997–1004.

49. Seible DM, Kundu S, Azuara A, et al. The Influence of Patient – Provider Language Concordance in Cancer Care : Results of the Hispanic Outcomes by Language Approach (HOLA) Randomized Trial. Int J Radiat Onclology Biol Phys 2021;111(4):856–64.
50. Shah RF, Mertz K, Gil JA, et al. The importance of concordance between patients and their subspecialists. Orthopedics 2020;43(5):315–9.
51. Meghani SH, Brooks JM, Gipson-Jones T, et al. Patient-provider race-concordance: Does it matter in improving minority patients' health outcomes? Ethn Health 2009;14(1):107–30.
52. AAMC. Fall applicant, Matriculant, and Enrollment data Tables. AAMC (2020) 2021.
53. Mankin HJ. Diversity in orthopaedics. Clin Orthop Relat Res 1999;362:85–7. PMID.
54. Aagaard EM, Julian K, Dedier J, et al. Factors affecting medical students' selection of an internal medicine residency program. J Natl Med Assoc 2005;97(9):1264–70.

Role of Health Equity Research and Policy for Diverse Populations Requiring Hand Surgery Care

Paige L. Myers, MD*, Kevin C. Chung, MD, MS

KEYWORDS

• Equity • Justice • Research • Surgery • Health equity • Public policy • Socioecological approach • Hand surgery

KEY POINTS

- Health equity is defined as eliminating systematic disparities in health imposed on marginalized groups resulting in negative health outcomes by allocating resources based on need. Equality refers to equal resources provided to all, regardless of need. True health equity cannot be achieved unless meaningful effort is applied to improve pervasive inequality.
- A socioecological approach can be used to evaluate the problems and propose solutions to health equity in Hand Surgery, specifically at the individual, community, institutional, and public policy levels.
- At the individual level, we must improve medical trust within diverse populations as well as providing patient education and strategies for risk reduction.
- At the community level, we must collaborate with community leaders to better help underserved populations. We also must invest in rural surgeons to ensure equitable geographic access to Hand surgeons and therapists.
- At the intuitional level, we must increase diversity and antiracist education of our workforce to better represent the populations we service. Institutions must increase collaborate to provide multidisciplinary, longitudinal care for vulnerable patients.
- At the public policy level, governmental agencies must thoughtfully collect data on all populations to assess areas of gaps and for progress. Through improve reimbursement and incentives from the Centers for Medicare and Medicare Services, patients with historically poor insurance can receive equitable Hand Surgery care.

INTRODUCTION

Public policy and health services research have meaningful impact on population health but can often have unintended consequences if the diversity of the population is ignored. Instead, policy and research should be viewed from the lens of health equity.[1] Although often used synonymously, equality and equity encompass two very different concepts. Health equity is an ethical principle driven by social justice which means that everyone has a fair and just opportunity to be as healthy as possible.[2] Equality refers to equal resources provided to all. True health equity aims to eliminate the systematic disparities in health imposed on marginalized groups that adversely impact outcomes.[3] (**Fig. 1**) Although there is a

Dr P.L. Myers has no disclosures. Dr K.C. Chung receives funding from the National Institutes of Health and book royalties from Wolters Kluwer and Elsevier.
Department of Surgery, Section of Plastic Surgery, University of Michigan, 2130 Taubman Center, 1500 East Medical Center Drive, Ann Arbor, MI 48109, USA
* Corresponding author.
E-mail address: paigelm@med.umich.edu

Hand Clin 39 (2023) 17–24
https://doi.org/10.1016/j.hcl.2022.08.002

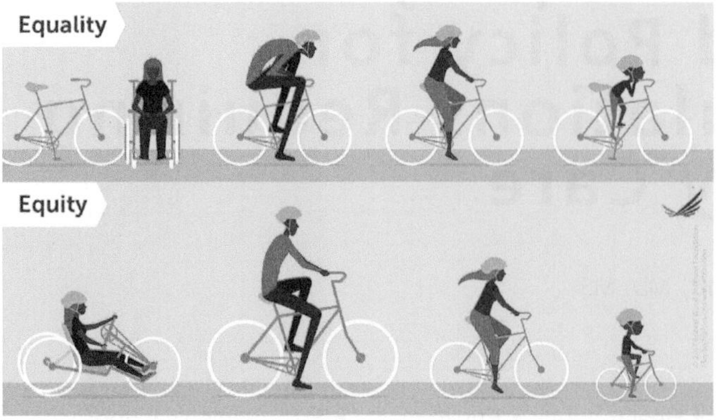

Fig. 1. Equality versus equity. To make meaningful change, we must not expect everyone to ride the same bicycle, but to ensure different bicycles for each person's needs. (*Courtesy of* the Robert Wood Johnson Foundation, 2017; with permission.)

well-recognized need to eliminate health care disparities, marginalized populations such as racial/ethnic minority groups, rural residents, and socioeconomically disadvantaged families continue to receive poor access and quality of health care. Despite advancements in medicine and technology, the persistent and ignored impacts of the social determinants of health undermine population health and wellness.

In a recent systematic review, research on the social determinants of health in Hand Surgery was sparse.[4] Race,[5] socioeconomic status,[4] and rural location[6] are all associated with poorer outcomes in surgery. Research in health equity and policy is essential for understanding the root cause, by guiding where to improve outcomes with an emphasis on implementing effective remedial strategies.[7] Chung and colleagues[8] outlined the intercalated relationship of research and health policy (**Fig. 2**). Research is necessary to describe a problem, policy is implemented to remedy the problem, and assessment is undertaken to elucidate the policy's impact and to refine the solutions. This cycle is repeated to offer the best outcomes for patients. In 1986, a national agenda for the Secretary's Task Force Report on Black and Minority Health was instituted to examine and improve health disparities. Despite this effort, there is still much effort to be made outside of the operating room.[7]

As surgeons, we are poised in a unique position to influence injustice. Conducting health equity research and with policy inclination strive to advocate for vulnerable groups. Factors such as social, environmental, and economic factors are pertinent to identify the barriers and propose solutions to achieve health equity. Despite thousands of published studies, our current knowledge is limited with regard to the most effective strategies to reduce health inequities,[9] though it is known that pursuing equity requires a collaborative approach engaging diverse stakeholders.[2] A socioecological model[10] conceptualizes the role of health equity research and policy for diverse populations in Hand Surgery. This approach considers the complex interactions among the individual, community, social, and political environments as it relates to health. It is useful for both understanding the nature of health problems as well as insight into the most effective methods for successful improvements by incorporating environmental change (not simply modifying individual behaviors).[1,11,12] We will be discussing Hand Surgery care for diverse populations through this modified socioecological approach that includes multiple levels: individual, community, institutional, and public policy (**Fig. 3**).[10]

INDIVIDUAL

At the individual level, there are biological and personal history[12] circumstances that contribute to

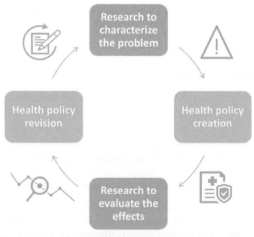

Fig. 2. Research is needed to characterize the problem, inform the development of evidence-based policy, evaluate the policy's effects, and guide policy revision. (*From* Chung and colleagues Promoting Health Policy Research in Plastic Surgery. Plast Reconstr Surg. 2021; 147 (5): 1242–1244; with permission.)

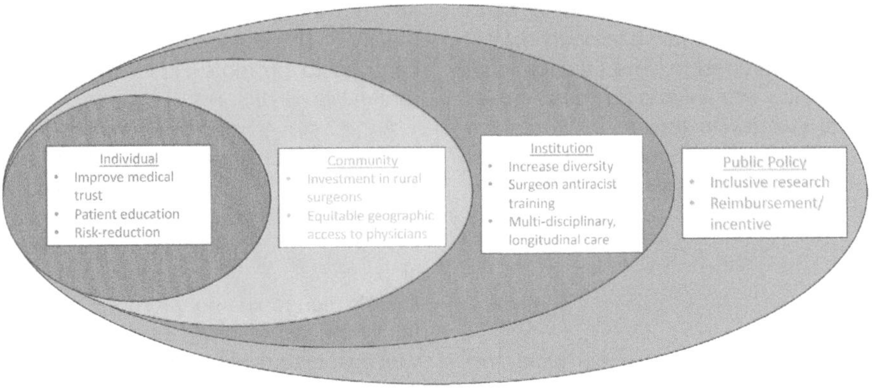

Fig. 3. A modified socioecological approach to health equity and research of diverse populations in Hand Surgery.

disparities in Hand Surgery care. One pathway that has led to this disparity is deeply rooted medical mistrust.[13,14] From Henrietta Lacks' cells to the Tuskegee Syphilis Study, there are many examples of how modern medicine has marginalized the Black community leading to reluctance to trust health care recommendations and seek care when needed. From 1932 to 1972, the United States government conducted a research study by forcefully denying incarcerated Black men proven treatment of syphilis to study the progression of the disease. The Tuskegee Syphilis Study is frequently cited as the most influential event precipitating Black Americans lack of medical trust, although it is not an isolated incident.[15] In 1951, at Johns Hopkins University, doctors obtained samples of cells from their Black patient, Henrietta Lacks, during treatment of cervical cancer without her knowledge or consent. These cells were discovered to have unique capabilities and were shared within the scientific community widely, still without consent. They have advanced the field of biology without any consent or compensation to her family. Ms. Lacks unfortunately passed away shortly after her diagnosis, never realizing her contribution. These are just a few examples of the systemic racism inherent in our health care system that has led to medical mistrust by minority communities.

To begin to systematically dismantle this barrier, Hand surgeons and policy makers can collaborate with community leaders to promote understanding of Hand Surgery care. This method has been proven successful in the past. In 2010, the Centers for Disease Control and Prevention launched the Racial and Ethnic Approaches to Community Health (REACH) initiative. This effort gathered coalitions of community health advisors, nurses, health care providers, and clergy to administer information regarding primary prevention strategies in African American communities. Through multidisciplinary collaboration, the REACH initiative successfully reduced disparities across the country. One example is increased screening for diabetes to improve awareness, prevention and control of the disease. In South Carolina, the hemoglobin A1C screening disparity between the African Americans and White populations decreased from 21% to 0%, and in Alabama, the disparity in breast and cervical cancer screenings decreased from 15% to 2%. This is important evidence that a community approach can be successful in reducing health disparities.[16] Even within our surgical practices, simply having an educated discussion can impact outcomes. In 2010, New York State passed the Breast Cancer Provider Discussion Law which greatly improved breast reconstruction rates, with the risk-adjusted rate growing significantly higher for African Americans and elderly patients.[17]

Hand and upper extremity trauma is the most common type of injury in emergency departments, responsibly for more than 12% of all trauma cases in the United States.[18] Currently, treatment of hand trauma is inequitably distributed. For instance, patients with hand amputation injuries who are African Americans, Hispanics, uninsured, or underinsured patient are less likely to undergo attempted replantation.[19] Patient comorbidities secondary to low socioeconomic status have more self-destructive behaviors such as greater tobacco use and unhealthy lifestyles can impact surgical outcomes.[20] Policy changes can be implemented to improve the safety of our vulnerable populations. For example, seatbelt[21] and helmet laws[22] have contributed to less morbidity and mortality from motor vehicle accidents, similar regulations can help minimize the burden of traumatic hand injuries. Gunshot injuries are a source of increasing injury with devastating effects.[23] Strict firearm laws can reduce upper extremity trauma for high-risk populations, clearly also improving the safety of the entire community. Fireworks are also an increasing source of debilitating hand trauma[24] that can also be curtailed through legislation on consumer purchasing. The Occupational Safety and Health Administration has implemented several policies to ensure to workplace safety for hand injuries,[25] although the burden of injury from occupational injury remains high, highlighting the need for even more work in this arena.[26]

COMMUNITY

At the community level, several geographic and socioeconomic challenges exist. The Emergency Medical Treatment and Active Labor Act (EMTALA) was created in 1986 to prevent discriminatory access to emergency medical care by requiring all institutions to accept emergency patients regardless of insurance status.[27] Despite this legislation, inequities persist.

For basic Hand Surgery problems, many community-based Hand surgeons do not accept Medicaid given poor reimbursements, which burdens patients to travel to a tertiary care center or safety-net hospital.[28–30] Complex upper extremity problems also often require transportation to subspecialists within Hand Surgery and/or a tertiary care center.[28] The disparity arises when patients with Medicaid insurance lack resources to travel and thus do not receive the necessary care they need or succumb to high out-of-pocket expenses.[31] Bias also exists in Emergency Medical Services transport, as Hanchate and colleagues[32] found that Black and Hispanic patients are more likely to be transported to a safety-net hospital emergency department (ED) compared with White patients within the same zip code. Long and colleagues[6] reviewed escalation of care for digital amputation and found that lower socioeconomic neighborhoods were associated with fewer transfers to a higher level of care, precluding these patients from replantation opportunities.

Rural populations also face limited access to health care. There are higher costs for travel to hand specialists with possibly more time away from work, adding greater stressors to the patient. The undesirable effect is the patient seeks care through nonspecialized physicians/surgeons or even ignores pursuing care.[31,33] Kalmar and Drolet found that geographic factors contributed to limited access to congenital Hand Surgery.[34] Rios-Diaz discovered that across the United States, there is a statistically significant paucity of Hand surgeons in rural and socioeconomically disadvantaged areas.[35] Establishing subspecialists in rural communities through policy changes may have great impact on health care equity while also providing economic growth for the rural community.[33] This research highlights the need for incentives to promote Hand surgeons to serve in rural America.

A recent systemic review outlined policy implementations to increase the health care force in rural areas.[36] An important finding emerged: retention of physicians was optimized by supporting rural residents training to the medical professions through local education, tuition waiver, and flexible schedules to promote employment and family needs. Simply paying higher incentives was associated with increased recruitment of physicians to rural areas, but low rates of retention.[36] Interestingly, the expansion of Medicaid and Medicare to rural areas disincentivized physicians, likely given the poorer reimbursements of these systems and the large proportion of the population covered by this insurance.[37]

Developing community–academic partnerships is a strategy that can be used to overcome these barriers. The organizations responsible for training Hand surgeons, namely the American Board of Plastic Surgery and the American Board of Orthopedic Surgery, can implement policy changes to better train Hand surgeons. There can be greater opportunities for training programs in rural locations as well as new fellowship models for rural surgeons to specialize into Hand surgeons during their practice. Through this model, the recruitment and retention of rural Hand surgeons can be maximized to better serve this marginalized population. In addition, larger institutions can invest in providing resources to these underserved communities to ensure they receive the care needed.

INSTITUTIONAL

Poor outcomes experienced by minorities are pervasive in the medical literature yet even surgeons do not recognize the problem—only 37% believe disparities exist, and even 5% in their own practice![38] All medical professionals—not just Hand surgeons—must learn cultural competence[39] and antiracist education[40] to serve patients, staff, students, and colleagues. The current literature is sparse and inconclusive on the most effective way to recognize and reduce implicit bias.[41] This will be an important area for increasing research efforts, though there are some strategies institutions can use.

The patient–physician relationship can be strengthened by greater diversity in Hand Surgery as patients feel connected by racial and ethnic concordance and improved care for underserved populations.[42,43] Increasing the diversity of Hand surgeons is necessary to improve health equity must begin in training. The most recent *JAMA* Graduate Medical Education Data[44] highlight this urgency for diversity in Hand Surgery. Of the listed training positions, 20% reported Asian, 8% Hispanic, less than 1% Native Hawaiian/Pacific Islander, and 0% Black ethnicities. Residency programs can be aware of the role of implicit bias in letter of recommendations and how this biased language may prevent an equitable selection process while also providing tools for avoidance of this language.[45] Our professional societies can establish formal pipeline programs at both the resident and medical student levels. They can sponsor scholarships for health equity research, establish diversity-focused visiting professorships, and formal health equity conferences to contribute to this cause. In addition, faculty members within Hand Surgery can support underrepresented minority students through mentorship and sponsorship to inspire them for Hand Surgery while also helping to improve their application to be competitive for the appropriate surgical residency.[46] A more holistic approach to medical student acceptance has also been shown to increase diversity in medical education.[47] Within higher education, focus can be given to deliberately teaching the history of the social determinants of health and structural racism to foster change in current practitioners as well as future generations.[5]

There is need for institutional improvement for preoperative and postoperative care of vulnerable patients. Occupational therapy is essential to achieving optimal outcomes in Hand Surgery, yet several barriers exist to access this important component of comprehensive hand care.[46,48] Zubovic and colleagues[49] discovered that after emergency department visits, uninsured and Medicaid-insured patients are significantly less likely to initiate hand specialty follow-up and to complete follow-up when already established with an outpatient clinic. This finding is multifactorial, though it can be attributed a lack of insurance with increased cost-sharing, poor health insurance literacy, geographic limitations, and lack of care coordination.[48] Another important study by Calfee and colleagues[28] found that patients with Medicaid insurance (26%) were significantly more likely to miss postoperative appointments than patients with private insurance (11%), with no-show rates increasing with the greater distance required to reach the specialist.

To ensure necessary follow-up, we can implement policy measures in all patient care settings, from the outpatient clinic to the operating room, and the emergency department. Automatic scheduling of follow-up appointments with telephone reminders, provision of transportation vouchers and waivers of fees at the time of the appointment are practices that have been shown to increase compliance rate to up to 80%.[50,51] In addition, strengthening interdisciplinary teams to include community primary care physicians, case managers and social workers can establish longitudinal episodes of care with less opportunity for patient attrition.[31] Patients will benefit from positive outcomes, including compliance with postoperative restrictions, management of comorbidities, and follow-up with hand therapy.[52] Prioritizing an approach of health equity can ensure that populations with the greatest unmet needs are effectively reached through institutional change.

PUBLIC POLICY

At the public health policy level, inequity manifests through several barriers of care for marginalized populations. Public policy interventions have the greatest impact against these barriers when they target socioeconomic variables, arguably the most impactful through federal legislation. The Affordable Care Act (ACA) of 2010 has led to the most significant changes for improving population health in the modern era, expanding access to health care to millions of previously uninsured Americans.[1]. It also established the Offices of Minority Health (agencies within the Department of Health and Human Services [HHS]) to allocate new resources to strengthen workforce diversity and to require nonprofit hospitals to collaborate with the community to conduct community health needs assessment This highligts the importance of a multifaceted and grassroots approach to health equity.

From a research and evaluation perspective, the ACA mandated that any HHS sponsored assessment include racial, ethnic, and socioeconomic demographics, the benefit of which provides more granular data, to better identify specific population health needs.[1] The literature has a lack of diversity of our research populations, and these data must be included to reflect our diverse communities.[53,54] One solution to ensure equitable research is to grow and link population-based administrative health records.[55] This data linkage, through advances in technology combined with racial and socioeconomic demographic data, can provide novel information for evidence-based health services research. Marginalized individuals often lack diligent primary care and may be more nomadic in their health care receipt, so by linking these records we can better track individual outcomes.

Despite the ACAs expansive coverage, many surgeons chose not to treat patients with Medicaid given poor reimbursement and burdensome paperwork requirements from Centers for Medicare and Medicaid and workman's compensation.[28–30,56,57] Targeted legislative changes should be implemented to increase the access of care to disadvantaged population through improved reimbursement. Further research is needed to characterize novel reimbursement strategies for Hand surgeons to include quality improvement efforts and by providing rewards and penalties as incentives to improve health care quality for the disadvantaged. In addition, more accurate indicators of surgical quality are necessary as metrics of success in Hand Surgery to emphasize more in the realm of form and function rather than mortality.

Reimbursement reforms may have unintended consequences, such as disenfranchising targeted populations or unfairly penalizing safety-net providers.[20] Billig and colleagues[58] outline a "pay-for-participation" strategy to avoid providing rewards to only high-performing, well-financed systems to mitigate the risk for further inequity. In this model, participants learn from one another and institute changes to improve patient care through quality. Such innovative methods focused on value are necessary as the US transitions from a fee-for-service to a value-based payment system. Reimbursements are increasingly tied to value, rather than volume. To evaluate the impact of policy changes on Hand Surgery outcomes, efforts should be devoted to assess value-based care through the lens of the social disparities of health.[8]

SUMMARY

Health equity ensures everyone has a fair and just opportunity to be as healthy as possible, despite unequal resources.[2] For diverse populations in Hand Surgery, a modified socioecological approach is useful for conceptualizing the role of health equity and research at the individual, community, institutional, and health care system levels. Collaboration among the community, policymakers, stakeholders, and health care professionals is necessary to achieve health equity. We must thoughtfully and willfully change the current practice to include these complex and multifactorial interactions within race, society, and the health care system. The quality of health care in the United States cannot improve until health equity is reached.

REFERENCES

1. Hall M, Graffunder C, Metzler M. Policy approaches to advancing health equity. J Public Health Manag Pract 2016;22(Suppl 1):S50–9.
2. Braveman P, Arkin E, Orleans T, et al. What is health equity? And what difference does a definition make. San Francisco: Robert Wood Johnson Foundation; 2017.
3. Hebert PL, Sisk JE, Howell EA. When does a difference become a disparity? Conceptualizing Racial and Ethnic Disparities in Health 2008;27(2):374–82.
4. Baxter NB, Howard JC, Chung KC. A systematic review of health disparities research in plastic surgery. Plast Reconstr Surg 2021;147(3).
5. Bailey ZD, Krieger N, Agénor M, et al. Structural racism and health inequities in the USA: evidence and interventions. Lancet 2017;389(10077):1453–63.
6. Long C, Suarez PA, Hernandez-Boussard T, et al. Disparities in access to care following traumatic digit amputation. Hand (N Y). 2020;15(4):480–7.
7. Woolf SH. Progress in achieving health equity requires attention to root causes. Health Aff 2017;36(6):984–91.
8. Chung KC, Baxter NB, Rohrich RJ. Promoting health policy research in plastic surgery. Plast Reconstr Surg 2021;147(5):1242–4.
9. Williams DR. Miles to go before we sleep: racial inequities in health. J Health Soc Behav 2012;53(3):279–95.
10. Golden SD, Earp JAL. Social ecological approaches to individuals and their contexts: twenty years of health education & behavior health promotion interventions. Health Educ Behav 2012;39(3):364–72.
11. Arcaya MC, Figueroa JF. Emerging trends could exacerbate health inequities in the United States. Health Aff (Millwood) 2017;36(6):992–8.
12. McCloskey DJ, McDonald MA, Cook J, et al. Models and frameworks. In: Silberberg M, editor. Community engagement:definitions and organizing concepts from the literature. Agency for Toxic Substances and Disease Registry; 2015. p. 20–3.
13. Butler PD, Morris MP, Momoh AO. Persistent disparities in postmastectomy breast reconstruction and strategies for mitigation. Ann Surg Oncol 2021;28(11):6099–108.
14. Musa D, Schulz R, Harris R, et al. Trust in the health care system and the use of preventive health services by older black and white adults. Am J Public Health 2009;99(7):1293–9.
15. Gamble V. Under the shadow of tuskegee: african americans and health care. Am J Public Health 1997;87(11):1773–8.
16. Airhihenbuwa CO, Liburd L. Eliminating health disparities in the African American population: the interface of culture, gender, and power. Health Educ Behav 2006;33(4):488–501.
17. Fu RH, Baser O, Li L, et al. The effect of the breast cancer provider discussion law on breast reconstruction rates in New York State. Plast Reconstr Surg 2019;144(3):560–8.
18. Maroukis BL, Chung KC, MacEachern M, et al. Hand trauma care in the united states: a literature review. Plast Reconstr Surg 2016;137(1):100e–11e.

19. Squitieri L, Reichert H, Kim HM, et al. Patterns of surgical care and health disparities of treating pediatric finger amputation injuries in the United States. J Am Coll Surg 2011;213(4):475–85.
20. Purnell TS, Calhoun EA, Golden SH, et al. Achieving health equity: closing the gaps in health care disparities, interventions, and research. Health Aff (Millwood) 2016;35(8):1410–5.
21. Prevention. CfDCa. Policy Impact: Seat Belts. 2011. Available at: https://www.cdc.gov/transportationsafety/seatbeltbrief/index.html. Accessed June 26, 2022.
22. Mayrose J. The effects of a mandatory motorcycle helmet law on helmet use and injury patterns among motorcyclist fatalities. J Saf Res 2008;39(4):429–32.
23. Meade A, Hembd A, Cho M-J, et al. Surgical treatment of upper extremity gunshot injures: an updated review. Ann Plast Surg 2021;86(3S Suppl 2):S312–8.
24. Morrissey PJ, Scheer RC, Shah NV, et al. Increases in firework-related upper extremity injuries correspond to increasing firework sales: an analysis of 41,195 injuries across 10 years. J Am Acad Orthop Surg 2021;29(13):667–e674.
25. Administration OSaH. Hand protection. 1994. Available at: https://www.osha.gov/laws-regs/regulations/standardnumber/1910/1910.138. Accessed June 26, 2022.
26. Duggleby L, Gourbault L, Parsons T, et al. How many acute orthopaedic injuries are preventable? Injury 2022;53(8):2790–4.
27. Zibulewsky J. The emergency medical treatment and active labor Act (EMTALA): what it is and what it means for physicians. Proc (Bayl Univ Med Cent). 2001;14(4):339–46.
28. Calfee RP, Shah CM, Canham CD, et al. The influence of insurance status on access to and utilization of a tertiary Hand Surgery referral center. J Bone Joint Surg Am 2012;94(23):2177–84.
29. Kim C-Y, Wiznia DH, Wang Y, et al. The effect of insurance type on patient access to carpal tunnel release under the affordable care act. J Hand Surg Am 2016;41(4):503–9.
30. Odom EB, Hill E, Moore AM, et al. Lending a Hand to Health Care Disparities: a Cross-sectional Study of Variations in Reimbursement for Common Hand Procedures. Hand (N Y). 2020;15(4):556–62.
31. Bernstein DN, Gruber JS, Merchan N, et al. What factors are associated with increased financial burden and high financial worry for patients undergoing common hand procedures? Clin Orthop Relat Res 2021;479(6):1227–34.
32. Hanchate AD, Paasche-Orlow MK, Baker WE, et al. Association of race/ethnicity with emergency department destination of emergency medical services transport. JAMA Netw Open 2019;2(9):e1910816.
33. Meyerson J, Shields T, Liechty A, et al. Creating a rural plastic surgery practice: social and financial impacts. Plast Reconstr Surg Glob Open 2022;10(5):e4293.
34. Kalmar CL, Drolet BC. Socioeconomic disparities in surgical care for congenital hand differences. Hand (N Y) 2022. https://doi.org/10.1177/15589447221092059. 15589447221092059.
35. Rios-Diaz AJ, Metcalfe D, Singh M, et al. Inequalities in Specialist Hand Surgeon Distribution across the United States. Plast Reconstr Surg 2016;137(5):1516–22.
36. Russell D, Mathew S, Fitts M, et al. Interventions for health workforce retention in rural and remote areas: a systematic review. Hum Resour Health 2021;19(1):103.
37. Zhou JT. Analyses of physician labor supply dynamics and its effect on patient welfare. Chapel Hill, NC: The University of North Carolina; 2018.
38. Britton BV, Nagarajan N, Zogg CK, et al. US surgeons' perceptions of racial/ethnic disparities in health care: a cross-sectional study. JAMA Surg 2016;151(6):582–4.
39. Baxter N, Chung KC. The plastic surgeon's role in health equity research and policy. Ann Plast Surg 2020;85(6):592–4.
40. Bradford PS, Dacus AR, Chhabra AB, et al. How to be an antiracist Hand Surgery educator. J Hand Surg Am 2021;46(6):507–11.
41. Maina IW, Belton TD, Ginzberg S, et al. A decade of studying implicit racial/ethnic bias in healthcare providers using the implicit association test. Soc Sci Med 2018;199:219–29.
42. Saha S, Komaromy M, Koepsell TD, et al. Patient-physician racial concordance and the perceived quality and use of health care. Arch Intern Med 1999;159(9):997–1004.
43. James SA. The strangest of all encounters: racial and ethnic discrimination in US health care. Cad Saude Publica 2017;1(Suppl 1):e00104416, 33Suppl.
44. Brotherton SE, Etzel SI. Graduate medical education, 2020-2021. JAMA 2021;326(11):1088–110.
45. Bradford PS, Akyeampong D, Fleming MA 2nd, et al. Racial and gender discrimination in Hand Surgery letters of recommendation. J Hand Surg Am 2021;46(11):998–1005.e1002.
46. Khetpal S, Lopez J, Redett RJ, et al. Health equity and healthcare disparities in plastic surgery: what we can do. J Plast Reconstr Aesthet Surg 2021;74(12):3251–9.
47. Grbic D, Morrison E, Sondheimer HM, et al. The association between a holistic review in admissions workshop and the diversity of accepted applicants and students matriculating to medical school. Acad Med 2019;94(3):396–403.
48. Krishnan J, Chung KC. Access to hand therapy following surgery in the United States: barriers and Facilitators. Hand Clin 2020;36(2):205–13.
49. Zubovic E, Van Handel AC, Skolnick GB, et al. Insurance status and disparities in outpatient care after

traumatic injuries of the hand: a retrospective cohort study. Plast Reconstr Surg 2021;147(3):545–54.
50. Messina FC, McDaniel MA, Trammel AC, et al. Improving specialty care follow-up after an ED visit using a unique referral system. Am J Emerg Med 2013;31(10):1495–500.
51. Baren JM, Boudreaux ED, Brenner BE, et al. Randomized controlled trial of emergency department interventions to improve primary care follow-up for patients with acute asthma. Chest 2006;129(2):257–65.
52. Vasan A, Hudelson CE, Greenberg SL, et al. An integrated approach to surgery and primary care systems strengthening in low- and middle-income countries: building a platform to deliver across the spectrum of disease. Surgery 2015;157(6):965–70.
53. Silvestre J, Abbatematteo JM, Serletti JM, et al. Racial and ethnic diversity is limited for plastic surgery clinical trials in the United States. Plast Reconstr Surg 2016;137(5):910e–1e.
54. Somerson JS, Bhandari M, Vaughan CT, et al. Lack of diversity in orthopaedic trials conducted in the United States. J Bone Joint Surg Am 2014;96(7):e56.
55. Hall SE, Holman CD, Finn J, et al. Improving the evidence base for promoting quality and equity of surgical care using population-based linkage of administrative health records. Int J Qual Health Care 2005;17(5):415–20.
56. Perloff JD, Kletke P, Fossett JW. Which physicians limit their Medicaid participation, and why. Health Serv Res 1995;30(1):7–26.
57. Malik AT, Khan SN, Goyal KS. Declining trend in medicare physician reimbursements for Hand Surgery from 2002 to 2018. J Hand Surg Am 2020;45(11):1003–11.
58. Billig JI, Kotsis SV, Chung KC. The next frontier of outcomes research: collaborative quality initiatives. Plast Reconstr Surg 2020;145(5):1315–22.

Advocacy for Diversity in Hand Surgery

Angelo R. Dacus, MD[a,*], Brittany Behar, MD[b], Kia Washington, MD[c]

KEYWORDS

• Allyship • Intersectionality • Pipeline • Concordance • Disparity

KEY POINTS

- Hand Surgery as a subspecialty has a lack of diversity in gender and ethnicity.
- The United States is becoming more diverse; however, medicine has not kept pace.
- Advocacy for diversity in Hand Surgery should start early.
- Diversity increases quality and innovation.
- Intersectionality involves overlapping identities in marginalized groups.

WHERE TO START

To know where to start in advocacy, one must first understand the "why" and understand that advocacy starts early. Although the United States is changing annually in several demographics, Hand Surgery is not. Although we are specifically discussing Hand Surgery as a subspecialty, we would be remiss if we did not note that Orthopedic and Plastic Surgery, which are 2 of the primary pathways to Hand Surgery, have failed to change. The concept of the "leaky pipeline" can be applied to Hand Surgery. This starts with limited exposure during medical school to surgical subspecialties, progressing through challenges in matriculation, compounded by disparities in program completion and academic appointment. Once training is completed, the leakiness of the pipeline is rounded out by low levels of senior executive mentorship and allyship, which make ascension to professorship challenging.

During the last 20 years, the United States has seen an increase in minority group populations reach beyond initial projections. Roughly 4 in 10 Americans identify with ethnic group or race other than White. The decade of 2010 to 2020 was the first in our nation's history where the White population declined.[1] Although the American population grows increasingly diverse each year, the physician workforce has failed to mirror this demographic change. In particular, certain medical specialties (eg, Orthopedic Surgery, Otolaryngology, and Plastic Surgery) have proven less likely to demonstrate significant diversity among physicians and surgeons.[2–5] Compounding the problem is the concept of intersectionality, which combines the ethnic disparity with that of an obvious gender disparity that also exists, with lower female representation in academic and surgical specialties.

Although women comprise approximately 50% of medical school graduates, they represent only 14% of Orthopedic Surgery residents.[6] African Americans and Hispanics comprise 13.3% and 17.6% of the US population but only 4.1% and 2.7% of Orthopedic Surgery trainees, respectively.[6] Furthermore, according to a 2010 study, there were 6.3 male applicants for every female applicant, 13.5 White applicants for every African American applicant, and 14.1 White applicants for every Latino individual applying to Orthopedic Surgery residency.[6] An article by Rao shows that the pipeline from residency to attending surgeons is leaking, with only 1.9% of current Orthopedic surgeons self-reporting as Black/African American, 2.2% as Hispanic/Latino, 1.2% as multiracial

[a] Department of Orthopaedic Surgery, University of Virginia, 2280 Ivy Road, Charlottesville, VA 22908, USA; [b] Department of Plastic/Maxillofacial Surgery, University of Virginia, 2280 Ivy Road, Charlottesville, VA 22908, USA; [c] Division of Plastic & Reconstructive Surgery, University of Colorado, 12631 East 17th Avenue, Aurora, CO 80045, USA
* Corresponding author.
E-mail address: ard6c@virginia.edu

Hand Clin 39 (2023) 25–31
https://doi.org/10.1016/j.hcl.2022.08.011
0749-0712/23/

and 0.4% as Native American.[8] The composition of Plastic Surgery residents and attendings is similarly lacking in diversity with no significant change in demographics of integrated Plastic Surgery applicants between 2010 to 2014 and 2015 to 2020. About 2.9% of all Plastic Surgery residents (integrated and independent) self-reported as Black/African American, 0.8% report as Native American, 11.7% as Hispanic/Latino, and 0.6% as Pacific Islander.[5]

Female representation among trainees has increased greatly but there has been a decline in Black representation of integrated Plastic Surgery residents despite increases in medical school graduates and applicants. The data highlight a discrepancy between the population of applicants and residents suggesting that barriers starting from medical school may contribute to the lack of diversity in Plastic Surgery.[7] Overall the field of Hand Surgery has had a higher female representation than the field of Orthopedic Surgery but below that of Plastic Surgery and significantly below that of General Surgery.[9]

Medical schools have a responsibility to expose students to surgical subspecialties and give students the opportunity to interact with potential mentors. Okike and colleagues[10] reported that musculoskeletal medicine courses in medical school have been shown to increase the likelihood that students will apply to Orthopedic Surgery residency programs, and the observed increases have been disproportionately large among underrepresented in medicine (UIM) and women. Increased exposure to Orthopedic Surgery can lead to the development of mentoring relationships and help to dispel potential negative perceptions of Orthopedic Surgery as a profession. By appealing to all qualified medical students, regardless of race or ethnicity, Orthopedic Surgery residency training programs can ensure that they attract the best and brightest applicants.

Across specialties, residency programs have reported using academic criteria such as United States Medical Licensing Examination (USMLE) scores, class rank, Alpha Omega Alpha membership, and meaningful involvement in research and extracurricular activities as important selection criteria for residency candidates. There is some evidence that using these criteria as residency interview screening tools may maximize training program outcomes such as first-time board certification success.[11] This unfortunately has put a perceived excessive emphasis on standardized testing as a measure of future success. This, in part, has led to the application of a pass/fail system for USMLE testing. Studies have shown disparities in Alpha Omega Alpha (AOA) selection as well as access to research opportunities among minority students.[12]

A study appearing in the *Journal of the AAOS* explored why members of racial and ethnic minority groups have a lower rate of acceptance into Orthopedic Surgery residency programs, resulting in a relative underrepresentation. The study revealed that less than 50% of applicants from black or Hispanic backgrounds actually enroll in residencies, whereas 69% of Asian and 73% of White applicants are accepted and matriculate into Orthopedic Surgery residencies. Underrepresented minority students comprised approximately a third of the applicants and less than a quarter of enrolled candidates.[13] Although several of the prior noted factors may contribute to these numbers, a study by Poon, and colleagues[14] found that ethnicity/race, but not gender, was associated with admission into Orthopedic Surgery residency, even when accounting for academic metrics.

ADVOCACY FOR DIVERSITY IN HAND SURGERY

Gains in diversity among Orthopedic Surgery fellows has plateaued despite initial improvement from 1995 to 2012.[9,15] Hand Surgery fellows in 2021 (both Orthopedic and Plastic Surgery) are composed of 2.1% Native American, 0.7% African American, 9.2% Hispanic/Latino, and 0% Pacific Islander. It is unclear what the diversity of the Hand surgeon work force is currently. Earp and colleagues[16] noted in 2016 that female surgeons composed 14.3% of the ASSH membership, African Americans 1.7%, Asians 9.8%, Hispanic or Latino 4.3%, and others made up 1.3% of membership among US members. A survey of Black Orthopedic surgeons in the United States showed that greater than 97% thought that racial discrimination in the workplace was a problem and less than 20% thought that Orthopedic Surgery society leaders were sincerely making efforts to end this.[17] Ethnic diversity remains lacking in academic Plastic Surgery groups with only 1.5% of academic Plastic surgeons identifying as African American and 4.9% as Hispanic as of 2004.[2] This unfortunately has not improved much with time with similar rates of diversity in the Plastic Surgery academic workforce in 2019 (1.9% African American and 3.5% Hispanic).[18]

Why Are Hand Surgeons from Diverse Backgrounds Needed?

Physicians and health-care professionals see themselves as “natural history scientists” who are immune to bias and always remain objective. This is despite volumes of evidence in the literature of patients' documentation of racial bias in health-care settings.[19] Simply increasing the number of traditionally underrepresented people in the workforce is not enough to counteract years of systemic racism, inherent bias, and worse health outcomes for ethnic minorities.[20] Antiracist interventions are needed to counteract this "blindness to race." These interventions can include focused multigenerational mentorship programs, purposeful actions to recruit, support, and maintain underrepresented minority and female surgeons within academia and the medical workforce and anti-racism trainings for physicians and staff across health-care systems.

Medical students who participated in mentorship programs that expose them early to surgical subspecialties are more likely to consider and apply to these for match. Successful programs, such as Nth Dimensions, are 14.5 times more likely to apply to an Orthopedic Surgery residency. This has also led to continued mentorship for underrepresented minorities in Orthopedic Surgery residency with focus on minimizing attrition rates and providing support through fellowship and attendinghood.[21] Nth Dimensions has been so successful that its model has been replicated for mentoring future dermatologists and Plastic surgeons.

Residency programs that lack diversity are unappealing to underrepresented minorities. Surgical residencies that promote gender and racial diversity through their websites, through outreach and through recruitment activities are more successful at matching and graduating female and minority surgeons. Ku and colleagues[22] show that females and underrepresented minorities value these activities when making their rank lists. Orthopedic and Plastic Surgery residency programs are lacking in these initiatives though. Examination of program websites and social media accounts show low rates of diversity, equity, and inclusion (DEI) promotion, of diverse faculty or discussion of DEI recruitment events.[23,24]

Continued mentorship and support through residency is critical to preventing attrition of female and underrepresented minority surgeons. In a survey of residents across accredidation council for graduate medical education (ACGME) programs, trainees who had thoughts of withdrawal from residency had significantly lower feelings of sufficient mentorship. Residents with ratings of neutral or negative experience had lower ratings of social isolation. Minority trainees had lower average scores for sufficient mentorship and higher feelings of isolation, along with more challenging execution of physician orders.[25]

HOW DIVERSITY IN LEADERSHIP LEADS TO MORE DIVERSE HAND SURGEONS IN GENERAL

Despite this, there has been an increase in the number of faculty members across Orthopedic Surgery institutions designated as the DEI department leader. However, there remains suboptimal support for this position, including protected time and funding, which limits the potential for change.[26]

There has been a small increase in the number of female authors from 2006 to 2019 in the Hand Surgery literature with an increase from 10.9% to 20.1% for first authors and from 7.6% to 14.2% in senior authors.[27] There have been some purposeful efforts within Hand Surgery associations to improve gender diversity and highlight female Hand surgeons. Directed efforts were implemented by the American Society for Surgery of the Hand (ASSH) to include women presenters in expert panels. A call for abstract and panel content at the ASSH meeting included strong consideration for proposals that include women, underrepresented minorities, and those from diverse practice backgrounds. This directed effort was proven to increase female authorship to 26% from 20% from the prior year. This also led to a decline in all male speaking panels from 46% to 29% from the year prior. This however did not affect female lead authorship after implementation.[28] Despite these gains, there are fewer female leaders in Hand Surgery leadership positions than would be anticipated (13.6% of available positions are held by women).[29] Hand Surgery fellowship directors are also lacking in diversity. About 13.3% are female, none are African American and only 2 (3.6%) are Hispanic.[30]

Using the business world as a model, we can see how integration of diversity into the leadership structure can reap large benefits to the field as well as our patient population. In a survey of more than 1700 companies examining diversity in management, it was found that companies with more diversity earned more revenue from new products and services, especially when women held greater than 20% of positions.[31] Inclusive workplaces show increased job satisfaction and engagement. Diversity reduces "groupthink" and enhances decision-making, with teams solving problems faster and producing higher quality intellectual property. Mixed gender teams also better manage team and group conflict.

HOW DIVERSE HAND SURGEONS LEAD TO BETTER PATIENT SATISFACTION

Racial disparities exist in health care even after controlling for sociodemographic variables. The previously noted meteoric rise in minority groups in the United States makes solving health-care disparities one of the most important aspects in improving our health-care system. African American patients are more likely to report that people of different races than them have different attitudes regarding cosmetic surgery and that a Plastic surgeon of the same race or ethnicity can better address their concerns and provide a more desired result even after adjusting for patients with higher income (above US$125,000 per year).[32] Patients report that physicians who share the same race as them report their visits as more satisfactory and lead to more patient participation.[33–35] Patients with a lower understanding of the health care system, a known barrier to patient satisfaction and outcomes, and is seen at higher rates in underrepresented minority patients, ask fewer questions during Hand Surgery evaluations.[36] Race concordant providers spend on average 2.2 minutes more with their patients, and patients seek physicians who are of concordant race with them, especially if they have had past experiences they deem racist with the health-care system.[37] Racial health disparities can be shortened through racial concordant physician–patient pairings, improving patient-centeredness communication, improving information giving, and focusing on partnership building and patient engagement during clinic visits.[38,39] Research has demonstrated that underrepresented minority physicians are more likely to serve uninsured patients and practice in underserved areas, leading to improved patient satisfaction and access to care for underserved groups.

Literature examining racially and ethnically diverse patients' utilization of total joint arthroplasty (TJA) are limited by disparate access to, utilization of and by worse postoperative outcomes. Racial-ethnic minority groups have worse preoperative comorbidities, are less likely to have private insurance, less likely to seek TJA surgery, and more likely to have longer postoperative length of stays or need skilled nursing facilities, and have increased postoperative readmission rates and more postoperative complications.[40,41] Surgeons are just as likely to recommend total knee arthroplasty to patients with clear indication for surgery for patients regardless of race or gender without high-risk comorbidities in simulation situations but retrospective data show that minority rates of total knee arthroplasty are lower even when adjusting for patient related and health-care system–related characteristics.[42,43] The Hand Surgery literature has a paucity of data documenting differences in access to and outcomes for racial discordant and concordant physician–patient relationships. This needs to be a focus of future research to better understand why a racially diverse Hand Surgery workforce is so critical.

DEFINING INTERSECTIONALITY

The term "intersectionality" was created by Kimberlé Crenshaw 1989 to describe the compounding social forces, identities, and ideologies through which power structures are legitimized. Initially, she used the term to discuss the exclusion of women of color from distinction in both the feminist and civil rights movements because of their dual identities, which essentially rendered them invisible.[44] Currently, the term is used to describe multiple levels of injustice for those with overlapping identities in marginalized groups. In reference to intersectionality in medicine, Balzora and colleagues said, "intersectional discrimination born from individual, institutional, and systemic racism and sexism is pervasive and embedded in the culture of medicine." Women of color who are UIM, in particular Black women, will be the focus of this discussion because they face some of the biggest ramifications of intersectionality in surgery and academia. Ignatius and colleagues[46] said "If true equality in the workplace is what we are after, sooner, or later we'll have to address the issues that are unique to women of color—and women of color and Black women, in particular in the workforce."

INTERSECTIONALITY IN ACADEMIC MEDICINE AND SURGERY

The Association of American Medical Colleges reported merely 0.7% of United States medical school faculty were Black women as of 2019. Furthermore, there were 60% more Black male full professors than Black female full professors, even though Black women physicians outnumber Black male physicians. Black women physicians are reported by the Economic Policy Institute to earn 27% less than their White male physician counterparts.[45] There are few Black women in academic surgery, and even fewer holding leadership positions. In fact, less than 1% of academic surgical faculty are Black women, compared with 49% White men and 14.5% White women.[39]

EXPERIENCES OF INDIVIDUALS WITH INTERSECTIONAL IDENTITIES IN SURGERY

Many studies have captured the experience of those from racial/ethnic or sex minority groups but there has not been extensive study of the experience of people with intersectional identities in academic medicine, surgery, and specifically

Hand Surgery. In a study of residents in training, residents considered sex or racial/ethnic minorities reported the negative impact of their identities on their training. In a cross-sectional national survey of 7409 General Surgery residents, 17% of respondents reported racial discrimination, and 32% reported sex discrimination. In a study by Samora and colleagues of female Orthopedic surgeons, 92% of respondents had experienced some form of microaggressions in residency or practice. Women of color are often omitted from dialogs and data in academic medicine, with the term "women" often referring to "White women," deleting the complex experience of women of color.[46] Recent studies of the effects of intersectionality in academia and clinical medicine have shown that women of color are more likely to feel unsafe in their workplace 40% of the time due to their sex and 28% because of race. Women of color are also more likely to experience racial harassment than their male counterparts of all races. They are equally as likely to experience sexual harassment as White women. The results of a survey of 274 Black Orthopedic surgeons in practice displayed the compounding effects that intersectionality can have on Black women. In comparison to Black men, Black women often reported a statistically significant trend toward diminished occupational opportunity and greater workplace discrimination. Black women also reported experiencing less inclusive and equitable environments and more microaggressions than Black men.[45]

While dealing with the challenges of racism, isolation, lack of mentorship, and unequal compensation, ironically underrepresented faculty of color take on the "minority tax," additional work which includes diversity efforts, mentorship responsibilities, and clinical responsibilities. Such service, although important, often does not meet traditional metrics for academic promotion and success.[47] A survey of attendees of the national women physician's leadership conference reported that nearly 50% of women physicians reported spending more time on service tasks than their male counterparts and a higher proportion of women of color physicians identified race as a factor in feeling obligated to volunteer for academic citizenship tasks.[17] Thus, women of color experience a woman minority tax in which they are expected to handle both minority and gender-related issues. Women of color from underrepresented backgrounds are often tasked with administrative activities, excess committee participation, handling minority and gender affairs, performing outreach and participating in media campaigns, and recruitment and retention of women and minority faculty.[39,48] The woman minority tax has also be called the "invisibility tax," and part of this experience can include Black women neither given credit for their ideas nor given acknowledgment for their hard work, which can lead to anger and resentment, and ultimately burnout.[46]

IMPACT OF INTERSECTIONALITY IN ACADEMIA AND BEYOND

The ramifications of intersectionality can take a toll on emotional and mental well-being. The internal fear of confirming negative stereotypes of a group is called "stereotype threat." Stereotype threat has been shown to have psychological consequences for Black women, including increased anxiety in health-care settings. Black women can fear being perceived as aggressive, bossy, and selfish when they voice their opinion when compared with White colleagues making the similar statements.[25] Moreover, Black women are more likely to be criticized and punished when in leadership positions. Black women can often think they are unable to be their authentic selves due to status distance, the distance from the perceived norm and power structure in an organization, which in the case of academic medicine would be White men. Ignatius and colleagues[46] states that "when you suffer from status distance, you'll seek to conceal status-confirming information about yourself... many Black women feel they have to dampen aspects of their personality to fit into the culture of their workplace."

SUPPORT OF INDIVIDUALS FROM INTERSECTIONAL BACKGROUNDS

Despite the challenges of intersectionality, underrepresented women of color have persevered and should be valued and supported for their resiliency, intelligence, and unique perspective. Improving the conditions for Underrepresented Minority (URM) women will undoubtedly improve conditions of other people with intersectional identities as well. Black women need to feel supported in ways that are specific to their background and experience.[25,49] The following are ways to support URM women: (1) Pay women of color equally to their White male colleagues; (2) Acknowledge the minority woman tax and provide monetary compensation for it and protected time; (3) Acknowledge implicit bias and implement ways to eliminate it; (4) Elevate and sponsor URM women; (5) Perform research that includes the experiences of women; (6) promote and protect URM women faculty; (7) Include people of all different backgrounds in diversity and equity efforts; (8)

Provide education and actionable steps to drive out systemic racism and sexism in academic medicine; (9) Learn to be an ally for women of color; and (10) Create an inclusive culture to avoid feelings of isolation for women of color. Steps toward justice and equity for URM women will ultimately make a better experience for all faculty improve the institution of academic medicine.

SUMMARY

A diverse Hand Surgery workforce is critical for the United States. Patients want to see physicians that mimic the population. The clear advantages are improved quality of care, an advanced variety of innovation, higher concordant patient satisfaction, greater access to care and improved compliance. Advocacy for underrepresented minorities and female Hand surgeons is lacking; however, an understanding of the data makes a compelling argument for change. This advocacy must start early in a surgeon's career, from medical school and continues through training and as an attending but it cannot stop there. Advocacy efforts are necessary to stop the progressive loss of diversity from early to more senior leadership roles. Hand surgeons who are both female and from underrepresented minority groups are especially vulnerable to bias from the health-care system. We must acknowledge the additional weight of burden they take on and provide them focused support and mentoring throughout training and their career.

DISCLOSURE

There are no financial disclosures by any of the authors.

REFERENCES

1. United States Census Bureau. National population by characteristics: 2010–2019. Washington, D.C.: US Census Bureau; 2020.
2. Butler PD, Britt LD, Longaker MT. Ethnic diversity remains scarce in academic plastic and reconstructive surgery. Plast Reconstr Surg 2009;123:1618–27.
3. Siotos C, Payne RM, Stone JP, et al. Evolution of workforce diversity in surgery. J Surg Educ 2019; 76:1015–21.
4. Ukatu CC, Welby Berra L, Wu Q, et al. The state of diversity based on race, ethnicity, and sex in otolaryngology in 2016. Laryngoscope 2020;130: E795–800.
5. Hernandez JA, Kloer CI, Porras Fimbres D, Phillips BT, Cendales LC. Plastic surgery diversity through the decade: where we stand and how we can improve. Plast Reconstr Surg Glob Open 2022;10(2):e4134.
6. Day MA, Owens JM, Caldwell LS. Breaking barriers: a brief overview of diversity in orthopedic surgery. Iowa Orthop J 2019;39(1):1–5.
7. Parmeshwar N, Stuart ER, Reid CM, Oviedo P, Gosman AA. Diversity in plastic surgery: trends in minority representation among applicants and residents. Plast Reconstr Surg 2019;143(3):940–9.
8. Rao RD, Khatib ON, Agarwal A. Factors motivating medical students in selecting a career specialty: relevance for a robust orthopedic pipeline. J Am Acad Orthop Surg 2017;25(7):527–35.
9. Bae GH, Lee AW, Park DJ, et al, ASSH Diversity Committee, Day CS. Ethnic and gender diversity in hand surgery trainees. J Hand Surg Am 2015; 40(4):790–7.
10. Okike K, Utuk ME, White AA. Racial and ethnic diversity in orthopaedic surgery residency programs. J Bone Joint Surg Am 2011;93:e107.
11. Dougherty PJ, Walter N, Schilling P, et al. Do scores of the USMLE Step 1 and OITE correlate with the ABOS Part I certifying examination?: a multicenter study. Clin Orthop Relat Res 2010;468(10): 2797–802.
12. Boatright D, Ross D, O'Connor P, et al. Racial disparities in medical student membership in the Alpha Omega Alpha Honor Society. JAMA Intern Med 2017;177(5):659–65.
13. Poon S, Nellans K, Rothman A, et al. Underrepresented minority applicants are competitive for orthopaedic surgery residency programs, but enter residency at lower rates. J Am Acad Orthop Surg 2019;27(21):e957–68.
14. Poon SC, Nellans K, Gorroochurn P, et al. Race, but not gender, is associated with admissions into orthopaedic residency programs. Clin Orthop Relat Res 2020. https://doi.org/10.1097/CORR.0000000000001553.
15. Poon S, Kiridly D, Brown L, et al. Evaluation of sex, ethnic and racial diversity across US ACGME-accredited orthopedic subspeciality fellowship programs. Orthopedics 2018;41(5):282–8.
16. Earp BE, Mora AN, Rozental TD. Extending a hand: increasing diversity at the american society for surgery of the Hand. J Hand Surg Am 2018;43(7):649–56.
17. Ode GE, Brooks JT, Middleton KK, et al. Perception of racial and intersectional discrimination in the workplace is high among black orthopaedic surgeons: results of a survey of 274 black orthopaedic surgeons in practice. JAAOS 2022;30(1):7–18.
18. Chawla S, Chawla A, Hussain M, et al. The state of diversity in academic plastic surgery faculty across north america. PRS GO 2021;9:e3928.
19. Hamed S, Bradby H, Ahlberg BM, et al. Racism in healthcare: a scoping review. BMC Public Health 2022;22:988.

20. Ely RJ, Thomas DA. Getting serious about diversity: enough already with the business case. Harv Business Rev December 2020;98(6).
21. Brookes JT, Taylor E, Peterson D, et al. The J. robert gladden orthopaedic society: past, present, and future. JAAOS 2022;30(8):344–9.
22. Ku MC, Li YE, Prober C, et al. Decisions, decisions: how program diversity influences residency program choices. J Am Coll Surg 2011;213(2):294–305.
23. Mortman RJ, Gu A, Berger P, et al. Do Orthopedic surgery residency program websites address diversity and inclusion? HSS J 2021;18(2):235–9.
24. Maisner RS, Kapadia K, Zhu A, et al. Diversity in plastic surgery: analysis of representation of sex and ethnic diversity in plastic surgery residency social media accounts. Ann Plast Surg 2022;88(3 Suppl 3):S257–65.
25. Aryee JNA, Bolarinwa SA, Montgomery SR, et al. Race, gender and residency: a survey of trainee experience. J Natl Med Assoc 2021;113(2): 199–207.
26. Taylor E, Dacus AR, Oni J, et al. An introduction to the orthopedic diversity leadership consortium: advancement of our orthopedic leaders of diversity, equity, and inclusion through networking, strategy and innovation. J Bone Joint Surg Am 2022;00(1–4):e1.
27. Xu RF, Varady NH, Chen AF, et al. Gender disparity trends in authorship of hand surgery research. J Hand Surg Am 2022;47(5):420–8.
28. Wessel LE, Pauslon AE, Graesser EA, et al. Moving the needle: directed intervention by the american society for surgery of the hand is effective in encouraging diversity in expert panel composition. J Hand Surg Glob Online 2022;4(2):65–70.
29. Brisbin AK, Chen GE, Smith BT, et al. Gender diversity in hand surgery leadership. Hand 2022.
30. Schiller NC, Spielman AF, Sama AJ, et al. Leadership trends at hand surgery fellowships. hand 2022. https://doi.org/10.1177/15589447211073977.
31. Lorenzo R, Voigt N, Schetelig K, et al. The mix that matters: Innovation through diversity. 2017. Boston Consulting Group.
32. Ligh CA, Lett E, Broach RB, et al. The impact of race, age, gender, income and level of education on motivations to pursue cosmetic surgery and surgeon selection at an academic institution. Plast Reconstr Surg 2020;145(5):932e–9e.
33. Cooper-Patrick L, Gallo JJ, Gonzales JJ, et al. Race, gender, and partnership in the patient-physician relationship. JAMA 1999;282(6):583–9.
34. Laveist TA, Nuru-Jeter A. Is doctor-patient race concordance associated with greater satisfaction with care? J Health Soc Behav Sep 2002;43(3): 296–306.
35. Street RL, Gordon H, Haidet P. Physicians' communication and perceptions of patients: is it how they look, how they talk or is it just the doctor? Soc Sci Med 2007;65(3):586–98.
36. Menendez ME, van Hoorn BT, Mackert M, et al. Patients with limited health literacy ask fewer questions during office visits with hand surgeons. Clin Orthop Relat Res 2017;475(5):1291–7.
37. Chen FM, Fryer GE, Phillips RL, et al. Patients' beliefs about racism, preferences for physician race and satisfaction with care. Ann Fam Med 2005; 3(2):138–43.
38. Shen MJ, Peterson EB, Costas-Muniz R, et al. The effects of race and racial concordance on patient-physician communication: a systematic review of the literature. J Racial Ethn Health Disparities 2018;5(1):117–40.
39. Bradford PS, Dacus AR, Chhabra AB, et al. How to be an antiracist hand surgery educator. J Hand Surg Am June 2021;46(6):507–11.
40. Chun DS, Leonard AK, Enchill Z, et al. Racial disparities in total joint arthroplasty. Curr Rev Musculoskelet Med 2021;14(6):434–40.
41. Mehta B, Ho K, Bido J, et al. Bilateral vs unilateral total knee arthroplasty: racial variation in utilization and in-hospital major complication rates. J Arthroplasty 2021;36(4):1310–7.
42. Dy CJ, Lyman S, Boutin-Foster C, et al. Do patient race and sex change surgeon recommendations for TKA? Clin Orthop Relat Res 2015;473(2):410–7.
43. Zhang W, Lyman S, Boutin-Foster C, et al. Racial and ethnic disparities in utilization rate, hospital volume, and perioperative outcomes after total knee arthroplasty. J Bone Joint Surg Am 2016;98(15): 1243–52.
44. Armijo PR, Silver JK, Larson AR, et al. Citizenship tasks and women physicians: additional woman tax in academic medicine? J Women's Health 2021;30(7):935–43.
45. Balzora S. When the minority tax is doubled: being black and female in academic medicine. Nat Rev Gastroenterol Hepatol 2021;18(1):1.
46. Ignatius, A. (Ed.). *How to Fight Racism at Work [Special Issue]*. Harvard Business Review. Harvard Business Publishing. August 11, 2020
47. Keshinro A, Butler P, Fayanju O, et al. Examination of intersectionality and the pipeline for black academic surgeons. JAMA Surg 2022;157(4):327–34.
48. Rodriguez JE, Wusu M, Anim T, et al. Abolish the minority woman tax. J Women's Health 2021;30(7): 914–5.
49. Williamson T, Goodwin CR, Ubel PA. Minority tax reform – avoiding overtaxing minorities when we need them most. N Engl J Med 2021;384(20):1877–9.

Recruiting, Supporting and Retaining Diversity in Hand Surgery

Micah K. Sinclair, MD[a,*], A. Bobby Chhabra, MD[b]

KEYWORDS

• Diversity • Leadership • Recruitment • Minority • Women • Orthopedic • Plastic • Hand

KEY POINTS

- Diversity and inclusion in Hand Surgery is necessary to overcome health disparities and inequities. All surgical fields that lead to a career in Hand Surgery have a stark lack of diversity of sex/gender and race, at every level of the workforce, from trainees to practicing physicians.
- Success in the development and retention of a diverse workforce requires sustained commitment from leadership.
- It is essential that leadership weaves the work of diversity, equity, and inclusion throughout all aspects of the work of the department or practice at the local level.
- Efforts to intentionally increase representation of women and racial minorities should be continued and encouraged locally, regionally, and nationally.

INTRODUCTION

> *"A truly inclusive corporate culture is one that accommodates all of the ways in which we are different from one another – and does so intentionally."* [1]
>
> *Ruchika Tulsyan*

The "business case" for the need for diversity, equity, and inclusion in companies has been established by multiple studies and researchers around the world.[2] The practice of medicine can be viewed as such; however, to view it solely as such diminishes the work that physicians do. Diversity and inclusion in medicine, and in particular, our field of Hand Surgery should strive to overcome health disparities and inequities. Without it, we will not reach equity in our provision of care.

All surgical fields that lead to a career in Hand Surgery have a stark lack of diversity of sex/gender and race, at every level of the workforce, from trainees to practicing physicians.[3–6] This continues to limit the pipeline of diverse Hand surgeons, due to the lack of role models and mentors for students and trainees considering their chosen career, specialty, and/or subspecialty. Additionally, it limits the education and professional growth of the current faculty in an inclusive environment that will benefit patient care.[1,7–9]

Although Hand Surgery has recently increased diversity compared with other musculoskeletal subspecialties, it still does not reflect that of our patient populations and studies on health disparities in Hand Surgery remains limited.[10–13] By improving the diversity of colleagues in our field, as well as all musculoskeletal care, we can improve doctor–patient communication and understanding of cultural views of health care, patient satisfaction, decrease health disparities, and potentially contribute to more physicians working in underserved areas.[6]

[a] Department of Orthopaedic Surgery & Musculoskeletal Medicine, Children's Mercy Hospital, University of Missouri Kansas City, University of Kansas Medical Center, 2401 Gillham Road, Kansas City, MO 64108, USA; [b] Department of Orthopaedic Surgery, Hand Surgery, University of Virginia Health, PO Box 800159, Charlottesville, VA 22908-0159, USA

* Corresponding author.
E-mail address: mksinclair@cmh.edu

Hand Clin 39 (2023) 33–42
https://doi.org/10.1016/j.hcl.2022.08.003

Although statistics on the low diversity in surgical fields are often published, a guide to effective recruitment and retention is lacking, and it is recognized that a single strategy cannot be applied to all.[5] The formula for change within one environment will be different than another based on the culture of each organization and the obstacles that are preventing the recruitment of diverse teams. The following information assumes supportive leadership and is meant to provide actionable items to consider based on publications and lived experiences, rather than serve as a prescriptive defined path to success.

Authors' Note: To narrow the scope of this article, we have chosen the audience of an academic leader. These recommendations can be formatted to fit any practice. Additionally, consistent with our culture to date, very few studies have been done to study the inequity of race. It is noted that the number of racial minorities within Hand Surgery, including Plastic and Orthopedic surgery, does not reach statistical significance in studies. This deficit is proof of the need for change.

RECRUITMENT

Commitment to Diversity, Equity, and Inclusion

> *"If you are neutral in situations of injustice, you have chosen the side of the oppressor."*
>
> *Archbishop Desmond Tutu*

Success in the development and retention of a diverse workforce requires personal commitment from leadership. Both your own commitment as a leader, as well as hospital and/or organizational leadership. Although your commitment should be inclusive of a mission statement, financial and time investments, you must also commit to supporting a change in culture of your department. This requires continual recommitment and the need to hold oneself and one's organization accountable. This is when the true change will begin and last.[1,9] Until our health systems and department leaders commit to changing the environment, it may unfortunately continue to be stagnant.

Create a Strategic Plan

> *"Diversity is being invited to the party; inclusion is being asked to dance."*
>
> *Vernā Myers*
>
> *"Equity is being part of the planning committee."*
>
> *Ruchika Tulshyan*

The commitment to recruiting, supporting, and retaining diversity in Hand Surgery requires a strategic plan, and along with this, cultural humility. To create the greatest impact, it is beneficial to elevate someone as a diversity leader to partner in developing the strategic plan and commit to seeing it through.[5] If your department or practice does not currently have diversity of physicians, consider contacting the Office of Equity and Diversity for your hospital, affiliated medical school, or hiring a diversity, equity, and inclusion (DEI) consultant. Do not assume that you are going to be able to solve this problem on your own. When creating a strategic plan, it is essential that leadership weaves the work of DEI throughout all aspects of the work of the department or practice.[14] This will aid in transformation of the environment to one of inclusion. If the plan is only to enhance diversity through increasing the number of diverse trainees and faculty/surgeons, without a commitment to changing the environment, the diversity will not be maintained. At each institution, the surgeon diversity leader needs to assess the learning and care environments, strategize effective interventions, and accurately measure the impact of change initiatives.[5] It is important to note that this change will take time and dedicated effort.

Strengthening the Pipeline of Future Colleagues

Improve diversity at leadership levels

Recent studies addressing sex diversity and work-family integration in Orthopedic Surgery noted a greater percentage of female residents in programs that had a higher percentage of female faculty, women at higher academic rankings, more women in leadership roles, and a women's sports medicine program.[15,16] Okike and colleagues reported that racial minority medical students who attended medical school at institutions with high racial minority representation among Orthopedic faculty and residents (>8% and >10.5%) were more likely to apply into Orthopedics than those with low racial minority representation among Orthopedic faculty and residents (<4% and <6.1%).[17] Multiple studies have confirmed the lack of gender and racial diversity in the leadership of both American Society for Surgery of the Hand and American Association for Hand Surgery as well as Orthopedic, Plastic and General Surgery departmental leadership.[14,18,19] This data provides an opportunity to understand our potential for change within leadership that can lead toward increasing the diversity of applicants, trainees, and colleagues.

Participation in programming is successful

"You can't be what you can't see."
Marian Wright Edelman

Successful recruitment of a diverse pool of candidates requires commitment to increasing the diversity of our trainees. Earlier exposure in medical school, mentorship programs, and trainee and faculty diversity can increase diverse applicants.[6,20–22]

Transformation of Promotional Practices

At the trainee level, one of the most important aspects of surgical training is the acquisition of skill through mentorship. The more we push aside those who need it the most, the more detrimental it can be to their skills. To combat this phenomenon, a surgeon must have awareness of one's own biases and create clear expectations and communicate these expectations to their trainees about participation in clinical care both in and outside of the operating room. Additional opportunities for skill acquisition, such as hosting industry laboratories or working with trainees in a surgical skills laboratory, can improve surgical confidence and enrich our participation as educators.

In addition to skill acquisition, research is another opportunity for mentorship. In creation of your DEI strategic plan, consider tying a commitment to education and mentorship of diverse trainees into the structure. An awareness that mentorship and education are a time commitment, thus with a limited number of women and underrepresented in medicine (UIM) surgeon mentors, there is a need for greater participation of all faculty in this work.

Once a department has hired a surgeon from a racial minority group or woman, the commitment to unbiased support, mentorship, sponsorship, and promotion must be a priority. This should include cultural humility, which will be discussed later in this article.

Ensure Equitable and Fair Salaries

Salary equity is a key component of an overall approach to equity and should be considered one element in a comprehensive diversity, equity, and inclusion strategy. Salary assessments are essential to implementing process changes that support equity, and should be evaluated at minimum at initial hiring, promotion, undertaking leadership roles and when creating an incentive structure beyond collections or the relative value unit.[23] It must also be noted that when considering salary audits, the data must be disaggregated.[24,25] The research of the Institute for Women's Policy Research has elucidated that "It will take 40 years – or until 2059 – for women to finally reach pay parity. For women of color, the rate of change is even slower: Hispanic women will have to wait until 2224 and Black women until 2130 for equal pay."[24] Of the women Orthopedic surgeons surveyed, 78% reported being the breadwinner in their home.[15] The cost of maternity leave is significant, thus there must be support given to change this. It devalues the participation of women and when they are already underpaid, which further contributes to salary discrepancy.[26] Finally, in addition to base salary, equitable compensation must also consider resources that are allotted to each surgeon, including clinical support staff, OR and clinic time, administrative assistants, and research coordinators.

Broaden Your Applicant Pool

To truly change the culture of Orthopedics, make efforts to mitigate bias in your hiring practices. Request referrals from a diverse group of colleagues and ensure that job openings are advertised publicly and broadly, including on websites of specialty group organizations that support racial minorities and women. Ensure that the duration of the job posting promotes a diverse pool of applicants. Plan ahead for anticipated retirements and growth to allow for a diverse group of applicants to interview. Although hiring practices commonly include personal referrals, consider that racial minorities and women often have less sponsorship, which translates to less potential options for employment. With regard to residency interviews, ensure that at least 50% of applicants are from non-White, nonmale backgrounds.

Holistic Application Review—It is Not Just for Residency Applications

"Endorse and employ a frame shift that challenges century-old ideologies that force minority populations to 'fit in' rather than belong."[7]
Bradford, DeGeorge, Williams, Butler

The holistic review process was shown to include a significantly higher than expected percent of female, traditionally UIM, first generation, and self-identified disadvantaged applicants in the interview pool than selected using academic metrics alone.[27–29] Create a consistent system in a holistic application review to combat bias.[30] If the process is not systematic, the inconsistency of your application review process can serve as a potential blind spot for bias.[17,26,31,32] Consider redefining what educational background you are seeking from your candidate. Recognize that different training programs provide variable opportunities for mentorship and scholarly activities. Ensure that you have a method of examining skills and intellect. Avoid interviewing only "those who you know are well trained." When checking their references, be aware of biased statements from your peers or colleagues.

Standardize the Interview Process

> *"Instead of wondering why they aren't thriving on the level playing field, imagine how the field can be changed to allow everyone to thrive."*
>
> *Emily Nagoski, PhD and Amelia Nagowski, DMA*

Through standardization of the interview process, it provides each candidate to have the opportunity to present themselves in a positive frame of reference. Seek to understand "How will this candidate enhance our culture?" rather than answering, "How will you fit in to our culture?" Create a corresponding interview scorecard with a rating scale and score immediately following the interview to avoid memory bias, where one is more likely to remember feelings and affinity rather than specific answers. If you cannot describe or are not consistent with the reason why a candidate is not a cultural fit, likely your consideration is biased.[33]

In preparation for the process, provide bias/allyship training for the selection committee. The traditional unstructured interview format used by many residency programs consists of open-ended inquiries reflecting the preferences and biases of individual faculty interviewers.[29] Unstructured interviews are heavily relied on in making ranking decisions, yet they demonstrate poor interrater reliability, low predictive validity, and unfavorable applicant reactions.[34] Through training for interviewers, mitigation of bias can be successful.

Support and Retention

> *"Increasing diversity does not, by itself, increase effectiveness; what matters is how an organization harnesses diversity, and whether it's willing to reshape its power structure."*[2]
>
> *Robin J. Ely and David A. Thomas*

Proactive Actions

The following actions provide a checklist of considerations to improve the DEI culture and initiative in your leadership practices. Unconscious bias is a key driver of leadership-linked disparities. Minority faculty have noted that they have experienced an inadequate recognition of work, exclusion from faculty activities, and alienation from fellow faculty.[18] Disadvantaged groups across the medical spectrum have called for improved transparency in leadership decision-making and the establishment of clearer faculty expectations for advancement.

1. Appoint and support a diversity leader in your practice.[5]

A committed faculty member to DEI work is of paramount importance. Include your diversity leader in the development of the strategic plan for the department. They must have decision-making authority, protected time for the work and a budget to support their initiatives and salary. Ensure that as the leader, you align with and support your diversity leader. This includes requiring engagement and accountability of your organization in addition to the physicians in your department.

2. Require education for faculty on bias, microaggressions, communication, and antiracism.[7,8]

Genuine and lasting change of an environment will require open minds and discussion about the team's personal growth in cultural humility. This ability for communication does not come easily, particularly when we have not been trained to communicate with our team in such a way. To facilitate this development, dedicated and protected time for education as well as facilitated content will best support lasting change. Expect that this is an iterative process and will take commitment and support over time to change the environment.

3. Be proactive and equitable in supporting and developing your faculty members.

Hold regular meetings with new surgeons—consider monthly and when comfortable transition to quarterly. Include a discussion of goals within the first few meetings and continue to revisit these goals at each meeting. Use faculty promotion or practice structure as a guide for goal setting to aid faculty in understanding opportunities for and deciding on their areas of career interest. This will aid in their identification of strengths and your ability to align opportunities with their strength and interest.

Ensure both mentorship and sponsorship of all faculty. Encourage mentorship participation equally throughout faculty. If it is incentivized, consider increased merit for successful mentoring of racial minorities and women, particularly at the trainee level. Evaluate everyone's ability to be a mentor. Simply calling oneself a mentor and being successful in this role are not the same. Recognize that mentors are not uniformly effective. As an example, when evaluating certain leaders for their mentorship, you may note that trainees experience great success working with them, leading to publications and successful match rates. At the same time, they may not be successful at retaining young surgeons, particularly women and racial minorities, in their division. Although a person may be an excellent teacher, he/she is not serving as a faculty mentor well. Expecting this will not necessarily lead to successful retention within the division. To retain faculty that work under such leaders, mentorship will be required through other avenues, such as other divisions within the department or departments in the hospital.

4. Perform annual reviews.

> *"Companies need performance management systems that tie feedback and evaluation criteria to bona fide task requirements rather than group stereotypes."*[2]
>
> *Robin J. Ely and David A. Thomas*

Provide consistent structure for annual review that is self-reported and allows the faculty to include accomplishments and future goals. Through these annual reviews, you will understand the work of your faculty and how you can support and sponsor their success toward promotion. If possible, meetings should take place in a neutral conference room rather than your office. Include intentional discussion about DEI work. To support accountability to your strategic plan and commitment to DEI work annually, at the conclusion of the annual reviews, collate the DEI work being done by everyone in the department and review it with the diversity officer. Consider it in the context of your strategic plan. Highlight publicly the successful work of others to encourage and promote further DEI work. Identify gaps and who may help to fulfill the work in those areas.

5. Be aware of the potential for bias within feedback systems.

If patient reported feedback is a part of the incentive structure, be aware of the potential for harmful bias. When providing patient reported feedback, it has been shown to be most successfully to share in 1-on-1 meetings rather than publicly posted and without comparison to named peers.[35–37] Understand the questions being asked of your patients, considering the patient's potential for unconscious bias to be involved in the score.

Include system level improvement work to support the feedback from patient satisfaction. Many of the considerations in the patient reported feedback are not under the control of the physician being rated. Attempt to equalize and elevate the ratings as a practice or department, rather than use the ratings to compare physicians to one another. If one surgeon shines, seek to understand how you can incorporate their success into the work of the department/practice. Through this, we elevate the care of our patients.

6. Be aware of the potential for bias in productivity models.

Concerning referrals, awareness needs to be paid as to how these are distributed. Depending on the payor model, evaluate the patient distribution to new partners. Often, they are assigned the Medicaid or self-pay patients. If your system includes collections-based incentive at any level, surgeons are disincentivized to treat these patients. An unfavorable payor mix can lead to lower collections, thus lower income for the young surgeon. Lower collections may lead to a false belief that they are not "doing the work" and therefore do not deserve a comparable salary. This may lead to earlier burnout of the young surgeons, which can lead to their leaving the practice or worse.[15,38–41] More importantly, this is also a discriminatory system that discourages care for the patients who are less fortunate and often need it the most. Be aware of gender bias against women surgeons. It has been shown that when the patients of women surgeons experience a complication, this can be detrimental to their referral stream. When it happens for men, it has much less impact.[42,43]

7. Support and celebrate all faculty successes publicly through use of internal websites and marketing.[7]

Create a relationship with the marketing department or director and educate them around your strategic plan. Ensure diversity in marketing, balancing the visibility throughout all physicians in the department, highlighting the work that they are proud of that is leading them toward promotion. If you are only celebrating that of the leaders who are established, this does not give the younger surgeons the opportunity to shine. Publicizing volunteer activities such as faculty involvement in activities aimed at developing a diverse pipeline for Orthopedic Surgery, such as the Perry Initiative, can both highlight the work of the department and educate the hospital system and community about the underrepresentation of women within Orthopedic Surgery.

8. Require leadership education for all surgeons.

Leadership is critical to our role as surgeons to ensure excellence in patient outcomes, clinical performance, and professional development. For success in the clinical realm, we must lead a multidisciplinary group of experts in complementary fields, including hand therapists, nurses, technicians, and administrators. Leadership skills are rarely intentionally taught within the medical, residency, or fellowship curriculum. The skills often overlap with those used for patient care, such as empathy, listening, and communication skills; however, they also include the ability for critical conversations, humble inquiry as well as strategic planning and alignment of departmental and hospital level goals.

9. Provide all faculty opportunities for leadership roles that lead to their advancement and promotion.

Ensure that you are supporting your faculty toward career advancement at the same rate, specifically by providing the same opportunities to women and racial minorities for leadership roles in your department, hospital, national organizations. Although achievements may vary, consider the mentorship that supports each surgeon to be successful at achieving their goals. If there is inequity of success, seek to understand what has led to this.

James White in Anti-Racist Leadership makes the point that men are often promoted on potential, and women and racial minorities are promoted only after they have proven many times over that they are deserving of the promotion. This he calls prove it again bias.[9] This statement emphasizes that the decision to apply, or recommendation to promote, often comes from a relationship with a mentor or sponsor. Consideration for promotion should be given to accomplishments and achievements when making recommendations. Moreover, if potential is used, this should be applied in the same way for all candidates, ensuring that the need to be unbiased has been considered.

10. Support each faculty through sponsoring their leadership in your medical school, hospital, and/or national organizations.

Ensure that you distribute the work among your group equitably. Having identified career goals through regular meetings, as well as knowing the strengths of your faculty, either self-identified or observed, will allow you to match each surgeon with work that will engage them and lead to success. If these roles are offered, ensure that you are clear about how much their time will be supported and they are not penalized for the time spent in their commitment to the success of the department.

11. Require Community engagement, both local, regional, and international for faculty on an annual basis.

This can include community "clean up" events, providing volunteer patient care at your free clinic, covering high school sports teams, supporting athletic events such as runs or walks, serving meals on holidays, participation in volunteer surgery with local or international surgical teams, being on the board of important local organizations. Include trainees in this work when possible. Consider engaging with the DEI office at your institution to understand opportunities for local impactful work that can be provided by the department.

12. Include articles at journal clubs that include health equity at each session. Host one educational session dedicated to addressing DEI topics annually.

With the awareness that care has been inequitable for non-White and nonmale patients, it is important to illustrate how this health inequity applies to the care we provide. This encourages our colleagues and trainees to consider bias in their own care and provide consideration as to how their own research initiatives and care processes may change to be more equitable. By organizing an annual journal club or retreat focused specifically on DEI, this can provide an opportunity to work together with skilled facilitators to aid in continued education and growth in understanding the inequity of our culture because it relates to patient care and collegiality. This inclusion of health equity research regularly will highlight the void of current antiracist research with the goal of inspiring curiosity and further research.

13. When developing a team dynamic—use validated and positive coaching and organizational tools.

There are several options available for workplace personality assessments, some more validated than others. Consider using the Clifton Strengths assessment test, developed by Don Clifton after asking the question, "What would happen if we studied what was right with people versus what's wrong with people?"[44] In medicine, this is antithetical to our mindset. We are constantly working to "fix what is broken" or how to solve the problem that our patient has brought to us. By taking an approach to building a team based on highlighting people's positive traits, it has been shown to lead to success. It is recommended that trained facilitator participate in the work for maximal improvement.

14. Have a family leave policy and clinical scheduling that is inclusive and fair for both women and men.

Flexibility and control over how teams accomplish their work must promote individuality, with the understanding that best practices must be followed, adequate access to care provided, equity ensured, and collegiality valued.[36,37] This is absolutely necessary when supporting work-family integration in surgical fields for this to improve gender diversity.[15,16] Regarding family leave for women, asking them to take extra call to "make up for their absence" while pregnant, needs to be reconsidered and because it may be a contributor to the higher risk of complications during pregnancy for women Orthopedic surgeons.[45] Similarly, we must also advocate for our male colleagues also to take advantage of family leave. In addressing these times of absence, if you or others experience bias around it, consider asking yourself or others what they would do if that surgeon had a medical emergency.

15. Ask that each faculty give a Grand Rounds lecture in an evenly distributed timeline to highlight their work. Consider inviting a diverse panel of visiting Grand Rounds or specialty series lecturers.

As Grand Rounds lectures are an opportunity to highlight the work of academic faculty, this is a good opportunity to promote the work of all faculty. In doing so, trainees can identify potential mentors within their intended or chosen field. This requires intention that there be a balance of speakers from the department, rather than simply the "senior speakers" from a group known to be majority White and male.[46]

16. Encourage research on health equity in patient care and require the consideration of health equity in every project.

It is essential that all patient populations be included in the research and quality improvement work done to support our patient care decision-making. Although this is often evaluated at the Institutional Review Board (IRB) level, understand that there is bias built into all systems. Seek to understand the diversity within the population that you care for and the resources of the hospital to support the participation of all patients in research. As with all fields of medicine, there is a great need and opportunity for health equity and health disparities research within Hand Surgery.

As health equity is understudied, consider encouraging younger surgeons or those surgeons with the most diverse patient population in the department to study their outcomes. Invite these surgeons to be the Grand Rounds speaker or on a panel at a national meeting. Ensure that they are participating in national registries. If this surgeon does not feel they have the time to participate, find ways to support them such as assigning a research coordinator or administrative assistant to their patient population to input the data into a registry or support a study. Allow them the time off to participate in a meeting, without penalizing them for this absence. When attending meetings with younger colleagues, introduce them to your peers to expand their network.

17. Incentivize accountability for DEI behaviors.

Require evaluation of diversity and inclusion efforts in performance evaluations. Link diversity and inclusion efforts to promotion of faculty to next levels of professorship. Use evaluation of diversity and inclusion efforts to help determine salary increases. Publicly acknowledge program residents, staff, and faculty who show inclusive values.

18. Commit to diversity of staff—in addition to faculty.

As a diverse group of leaders is important, so is a diverse team. By encouraging inclusive hiring practices in your clinics and operating rooms and with the appropriate leadership of these staff, will aid in changing the environment and culture. Middle management, such as clinic or operating room management, is of key importance to this cultural change.[9] Because they are the leaders of your staff, it will be important to partner with them, and the hospital system, on this initiative.

REACTIVE ACTIONS

1. Resist personal bias and use a process of due diligence when reacting to concerns or complaints about all faculty, especially racial minorities, and women.

Having a preestablished relationship with each faculty member, which includes regular meetings, annual reviews, routine feedback from residents, and staff who work directly with that faculty member, leads to improvement for each person. When necessary, it will aid in avoiding a negative bias toward the faculty when negative reports are made. Remember that all leaders make mistakes. Consider each situation with a root cause analysis, using due diligence to understand the occurrence. Most often, these arise due to miscommunication and with bias involved. Several studies have noted that racial minority and female trainees contending with discrimination and less respect than their peers often feel that they are less valued or underappreciated. This has been shown to lead to attrition and burnout in the trainee population.[4,17,22] If due diligence is truly used to understand the reported concern, and the consideration given to the potential for multiple biases in the interaction, this may lead to culture change that retains diverse faculty members.

2. Pulse check human resources (HR) by evaluating the complaints and interactions that have occurred around racial minorities and women.

Multiple important studies have evaluated discrimination of surgeons in the workplace.[4,41,47] Sudol and colleagues confirmed the association among racial/ethnic–minority surgeons and anesthesiologists with a high risk of discrimination and mistreatment.[47] Women surgeons in all specialties were found to experience a gender-based double standard in their conflicts, due to an expectation that they conform to gender over professional norms. The authors recognized the need for equitable adjudication of conflicts to lead to a change in their work environment.[48] By discussing these concerns with HR, it may allow for identification of systemic gaps in bias that can be addressed. This may be a role for an ombudsperson within the institution.

3. Create a supportive structure for faculty when they have surgical complications.

Surgical complications and litigation can be some of the most stressful times in our career. For women and racial minorities, this may compound to an already stressful environment and can lead to feelings of isolation. Many departments have a process for reviewing these cases internally. Yet, a well-established system for the faculty member to process their own stress from the event and subsequent management of it does not exist to our knowledge, other than individuals who independently seek counseling. Consider meeting with these surgeons and supporting them through the process when appropriate. If you see a change in their productivity, consider the potential for a change in referral patterns as a result and provide an avenue for support.[43]

4. Recognize signs of physician burnout and support faculty to avoid this or recover if they are experiencing it.

It is important to recognize that burnout can lead to increased complications and perceived disruptive physician behavior.[39] Orthopedics overall have recently been found to have a higher prevalence of suicide.[40,41] Prior literature has also shown that female surgeons experience dissatisfaction with the ability to maintain relationships with family and the ability to parent, and this is associated with higher levels of burnout, depression, and low career satisfaction.[15,42] Thus given the high potential for burnout and isolation in women and racial minority faculty, leaders must recognize, understand, and address the unique challenges of their underrepresented employees that can lead to a downward spiral and subsequent attrition.[22,49]

SUMMARY

> *"...I believe deeply that we cannot solve the challenges of our time unless we solve them together, ... by understanding that we may have different stories, but we hold common hopes; that we may not look the same and we may not have come from the same place, but we all want to move in the same direction – toward a better future for our children and our grandchildren."*
>
> *Barack Obama*

This work is collection of considerations for the work that we all must do, rather than a defined recipe to success. There is no "one size fits all" solution. Our expectation is that as our culture begins to change, so will the process. We look forward to hearing your experiences and all that is learned in the process.

CONFLICTS OF INTEREST

No conflicts of interest or funding sources.

REFERENCES

1. Inclusion on Purpose: an Intersectional approach to creating a culture of belonging at work – Ruchika Tulshyan61. Cambridge, Massachusetts & London, England: The MIT Press; 2022.

2. Ely RJ, Thomas DA. Getting Serious About Diversity: Enough Already with the Business Case. Harv Bus Rev 2020;November-December.
3. Hall JA, Chen W, Bhayana K, et al. Quantifying the Pipeline of Ethnically Underrepresented in Medicine Physicians in Academic Plastic Surgery Leadership. Ann Plast Surg 2021;87(4):e51–61.
4. Ode GE, Brooks JT, Middleton KK, et al. Perception of Racial and Intersectional Discrimination in the Workplace Is High Among Black Orthopaedic Surgeons: Results of a Survey of 274 Black Orthopaedic Surgeons in Practice. J Am Acad Orthop Surg 2022;30(1):7–18.
5. Taylor E, Dacus AR, Oni J, et al. An Introduction to the Orthopaedic Diversity Leadership Consortium: Advancement of Our Orthopaedic Leaders of Diversity, Equity, and Inclusion Through Networking, Strategy, and Innovation. J Bone Joint Surg Am 2022. https://doi.org/10.2106/JBJS.21.01350.
6. Harrington MA, Rankin EA, Ladd AL, et al. The Orthopaedic Workforce Is Not as Diverse as the Population It Serves: Where Are the Minorities and the Women?: AOA Critical Issues Symposium. J Bone Joint Surg Am 2019;101(8):e31.
7. Bradford PS, Dacus AR, Chhabra AB, et al. How to Be An Antiracist Hand Surgery Educator. J Hand Surg Am 2021;46(6):507–11.
8. Bradford PS, DeGeorge BR Jr, Williams SH, et al. How to Embrace Antiracism as a US Plastic Surgeon: Definitions, Principles, and Practice. Plast Reconstr Surg Glob Open 2020;8(9):e3185.
9. Anti-Racist Leadership. How to Transform a corporate culture in a race-Conscious world – James D white with Krista white. Harvard Business Review Press; 2022.
10. Khetpal S, Lopez J, Redett RJ, et al. Health Equity and Healthcare Disparities in Plastic Surgery: What We Can Do. J Plast Reconstr Aesthet Surg 2021; 74(12):3251–9.
11. Kalliainen LK, Wisecarver I, Cummings A, et al. Sex Bias in Hand Surgery Research. J Hand Surg Am 2018;43(11):1026–9.
12. Brisbin AK, Chen W, Goldschmidt E, et al. Gender Diversity in Hand Surgery Leadership. Hand (N Y). 2022. https://doi.org/10.1177/15589447211038679.
13. Surawicz CM. Women in Leadership: Why So Few and What to Do About It. J Am Coll Radiol 2016; 13(12 Pt A):1433–7.
14. Institute of Women's Policy Research (IWPR). Pay equity and discrimination. 2021. Available at: https://iwpr.org/equal-pay-about/. Accessed July 27, 2021.
15. Ponzio DY, Bell C, Stavrakis A, et al. Discrepancies in Work-Family Integration Between Female and Male Orthopaedic Surgeons. J Bone Joint Surg Am 2022;104(5):465–72.
16. Sobel AD, Cox RM, Ashinsky B, et al. Analysis of factors related to the sex diversity in orthopaedic residency programs in the United States. J Bone Joint Surg Am 2018;100(11):e79.
17. Ode GE, Bradford L, Ross WA Jr, et al. Achieving a Diverse, Equitable, and Inclusive Environment for the Black Orthopaedic Surgeon: Part 1: Barriers to Successful Recruitment of Black Applicants. J Bone Joint Surg Am 2021;103(3):e9.
18. Smith BT, Egro FM, Murphy CP, et al. An Evaluation of Race Disparities in Academic Plastic Surgery. Plast Reconstr Surg 2020;145(1):268–77.
19. Schiller NC, Spielman AF, Sama AJ, et al. Leadership Trends at Hand Surgery Fellowships. Hand (N Y) 2022. https://doi.org/10.1177/15589447211073977.
20. Okike K, Phillips DP, Johnson WA, et al. Orthopaedic Faculty and Resident Racial/Ethnic Diversity is Associated With the Orthopaedic Application Rate Among Underrepresented Minority Medical Students. J Am Acad Orthop Surg 2020;28(6):241–7.
21. Buckley J, Dearolf L, Lattanza L. The Perry Initiative: Building the Pipeline for Women in Orthopaedics. J Am Acad Orthop Surg 2022;30(8):358–63.
22. Aryee JNA, Bolarinwa SA, Montgomery SR Jr, et al. Race, Gender, and Residency: a Survey of Trainee Experience. J Natl Med Assoc 2021;113(2):199–207.
23. Dandar VM, Lautenberger DM, Garrison G. Exploring faculty salary equity at U.S. medical schools by gender and race/ethnicity. Washington, DC: Association of American Medical Colleges; 2021. Available at: https://www.aamc.org/data-reports/workforce/report/exploring-faculty-salary-equity-us -medical-schools-gender-and-race/ethnicity.
24. Ly DP, Seabury SA, Jena AB. Differences in incomes of physicians in the United States by race and sex: observational study. BMJ 2016;353:i2923.
25. Gottlieb AS, Jagsi R. Closing the Gender Pay Gap in Medicine. N Engl J Med 2021;385(27):2501–4.
26. Poon S, Nellans K, Rothman A, et al. Underrepresented Minority Applicants Are Competitive for Orthopaedic Surgery Residency Programs, but Enter Residency at Lower Rates. J Am Acad Orthop Surg 2019;27(21):e957–68.
27. Mason BS, Ross W, Chambers MC, et al. Pipeline program recruits and retains women and underrepresented minorities in procedure-based specialties: A brief report. Am J Surg 2017;213(4):662–5.
28. Llado-Farrulla M, Fosnot J, Couto J, et al. In Search of Workforce Diversity? A Program's Successful Approach. Plast Reconstr Surg 2021;147(5):1229–33.
29. Association of American Medical Colleges' Roadmap to Diversity: Integrating holistic review practices into medical school admission processes. Available at: https://members.aamc.org/eweb/upload/Roadmap%20to%20Diversity%20Integrating%20.Holistic%20.Review.pdf
30. Capers Q, Clinchot D, McDougle L, et al. Implicit racial bias in medical school admissions. Acad Med 2017;92(3):365–9.

31. Poon SC, Nellans K, Gorroochurn P, et al. Race, But Not Gender, Is Associated with Admissions into Orthopaedic Residency Programs. Clin Orthop Relat Res 2020. https://doi.org/10.1097/CORR.0000000000001553.
32. Bradford PS, Akyeampong D, Fleming MA 2nd, et al. Racial and Gender Discrimination in Hand Surgery Letters of Recommendation. J Hand Surg Am 2021;46(11):998–1005. e2.
33. Available at: https://biasinterrupters.org/
34. Grabowski CJ. Impact of holistic review on student interview pool diversity. Adv Health Sci Educ Theory Pract 2018;23(3):487–98. https://doi.org/10.1007/s10459-017-9807-9.
35. Vilendrer SM, Kling SMR, Wang H, et al. How Feedback Is Given Matters: A Cross-Sectional Survey of Patient Satisfaction Feedback Delivery and Physician Well-being. Mayo Clin Proc 2021;96(10):2615–27.
36. Shanafelt TD, Noseworthy JH. Executive Leadership and Physician Well-being: Nine Organizational Strategies to Promote Engagement and Reduce Burnout. Mayo Clin Proc 2017;92(1):129–46.
37. Shanafelt T, Trockel M, Rodriguez A, et al. Wellness-Centered Leadership: Equipping Health Care Leaders to Cultivate Physician Well-Being and Professional Fulfillment. Acad Med 2021;96(5):641–51.
38. Brown SD, Goske MJ, Johnson CM. Beyond substance abuse: stress, burnout, and depression as causes of physician impairment and disruptive behavior. J Am Coll Radiol 2009;6(7):479, 85PMID.
39. Jennings JM, Gold PA, Nellans K, et al. Orthopaedic Surgeons Have a High Prevalence of Burnout, Depression, and Suicide: Review of Factors Which Contribute or Reduce Further Harm. J Am Acad Orthop Surg 2022;30(5):e528–35.
40. Stein MK, Fryhofer GW, Blumenthal S, et al. Behavior in Orthopaedics Over Mental Health (BOOM) Group. Objects in Mirror Are Closer Than They Appear: Symptoms of Depression and Suicidality in Orthopaedic Surgeons. J Bone Joint Surg Am 2022;104(11):959–70.
41. Ames SE, Cowan JB, Kenter K, et al. Burnout in Orthopaedic Surgeons: A Challenge for Leaders, Learners, and Colleagues: AOA Critical Issues. J Bone Joint Surg Am 2017;99(14):e78.
42. Women surgeons are punished more than men for the exact same mistakes, study finds - VOX 2017
43. Finnegan J. Women surgeons pay tougher consequences than male colleagues for bad health outcomes. Fierce Healthc 2017. Available at: https://www.fiercehealthcare.com/practices/gender-plays-part-surgeon-referrals-heather-sarsons-harvard.
44. Available at: https://www.gallup.com/cliftonstrengths/en/252137/home.aspx?utm_source=google&utm_medium=cpc&utm_campaign=us_strengths_branded_cs_ecom&utm_term=clifton%20strengths%20assessment&gclid=EAIaIQobChMImK-Hm8uW-AIVkWxvBB3qSQFkEAAYASAAEgKv-PD_BwE.
45. Poon S, Luong M, Hargett D, et al. Does a Career in Orthopaedic Surgery Affect a Woman's Fertility? J Am Acad Orthop Surg 2021;29(5):e243–50.
46. Boiko JR, Anderson AJM, Gordon RA. Representation of Women Among Academic Grand Rounds Speakers. JAMA Intern Med 2017;177(5):722–4.
47. Sudol NT, Guaderrama NM, Honsberger P, et al. Prevalence and Nature of Sexist and Racial/Ethnic Microaggressions Against Surgeons and Anesthesiologists. JAMA Surg 2021;156(5):e210265.
48. Dossett LA, Vitous CA, Lindquist K, et al. Women Surgeons' Experiences of Interprofessional Workplace Conflict. JAMA Netw Open 2020;3(10):e2019843.
49. Hu YY, Ellis RJ, Hewitt DB, et al. Discrimination, Abuse, Harassment, and Burnout in Surgical Residency Training. N Engl J Med 2019;381(18):1741–52.

Inclusive Mentorship and Sponsorship

Kamali Thompson, MD, MBA[a], Erica Taylor, MD, MBA[b,*]

KEYWORDS

• Inclusive Mentorship • Sponsorship • Hand Surgery • Diversity • Equity • Inclusion

KEY POINTS

- Barriers to inclusive mentorship center upon the current mindset of prospective mentors and potential obstacles to building a relationship with a mentee of a different background.
- Specific barriers fall into six categories: (1) traditional views of success, (2) lack of validation, (3) focus on rescue, (4) diminished value of achievements, (5) mixed goal agreement, and (6) mixed motivations.
- Solution-based approaches must be accepted by the medical community to bridge gaps within the surgical field and form inclusive mentoring relationships.
- The medical community can look to pioneering organizations that have leaned into the complex work of diversity, equity, and inclusion for additional support, insight, and resources.

THE EVOLUTION OF MENTORSHIP

Mentorship, which is simplistically defined as the process of guidance being passed from one individual with more experience to another with less experience, has been considered a core component across all our medical and surgical specialties. Its roots are often traced to the character of Mentor in the Odyssey (Homer), a text that details Odysseus' perilous journey following the Trojan War. In this narrative, the old friend Mentor appears and provides support and guidance during various trials of the plot. Fast forward centuries later, the art of mentoring—and the critical need for mentorship—continues to exist today as a central aspect of one's own personal and professional success.

One can only imagine the challenges faced by Odysseus and his family are not the same as the workplace or academic needs that warrant intentional mentorship today. That said, the principles are similar. Over the last several decades, we have watched mentorship evolve from an organic connection between two individuals who may share similar goals, vision, interests, or assignments, to a more structured process that was initially assigned in the workplace to help certain groups become aware and accustomed to professional politics. As the concept of mentoring spread to a more universal approach, with medical students, trainees, and faculty all being asked to identify mentors, we have seen the term "mentorship" being used with so much regularity that even Odysseus himself would be shocked. In fact, in academic settings and societies, awards are given to recognize the best mentors and faculty promotion decisions consider how many individuals a candidate for promotion has mentored over his/her tenure. Accordingly, we have seen an increase in individuals desiring mentors across all medical professional designations, as well as a rise in individuals seeking to become mentors to others. As a byproduct, often touted as the next step to mentorship, sponsorship also became popularized as the next phase. The goal of sponsorship has been to take the benefits of mentorship (guidance) into the decision-making environments (advocacy) to promote and publicly support the mentee. One adage is that sponsorship is bringing someone into a room, figuratively, without them having to be there.

The authors have nothing to disclose.
[a] Temple University Hospital, Philadelphia, PA, USA; [b] Duke University School of Medicine, PO Box 1726, Wake Forest, NC 27587, USA
* Corresponding author.
E-mail address: erica.taylor@duke.edu

Hand Clin 39 (2023) 43–52
https://doi.org/10.1016/j.hcl.2022.08.012
0749-0712/23/

With that amount of attention, there is controversy over whether mentorship is truly organic and intrinsic, or if it should be constructed and manufactured. *Is one born a mentor? Does everyone need a mentor? What makes a "good" mentor?* Many have explored, and postulated, various criteria for effective mentoring, including knowledge in the subject matter, proven success, benevolence, directness, and communication skills (including an ability to listen). Considering the potential impact mentorship and sponsorship can have on personal and professional experiences, it is important to execute them with care so that the results of these touchpoints are positive and productive. However, what has not be readily explored and promoted, is the importance of *inclusive mentoring.* We have asked, *is mentorship available to everyone in the same quantity and the same quality? If not, why not?* In this article, we will dive deeper into the concept of inclusive mentorship and sponsorship, and their inextricable link to areas of diversity, equity, and inclusion in our professions. We will set the stage using Orthopedic Surgery as the example field, given its designation as one of the least diverse medical specialties with extremely low numbers of female and minority resident, fellows, and attendings despite decades of efforts. Inclusive mentorship and sponsorship provide the opportunity to bridge these gaps.

MENTORSHIP AND SPONSORSHIP IN THE TWENTY-FIRST CENTURY

The concept of mentorship has been in existence for centuries and is accepted into the academic zeitgeist as a core principle and offering to learners and faculty. As entry into medical school, residency, fellowship, and the job market become more competitive, applicants look for guidance to enhance their chances to achieve their goals. This has resulted in the establishment of many formal mentoring programs and has increased the popularity of individual one-on-one mentorship. Furthermore, students with less experience or resources in the medical field are theoretically provided an opportunity to reach an even playing field with their counterparts with this guidance from more experienced individuals who have reached a certain stage of achievement.

Guidance and advocacy come in various formats. The advent of the internet and social media has expanded the possibilities, resulting in greater reach and visibility. When students in the high school, college, and medical school phases can see themselves represented by aspirational figures, and can communicate with or follow these individuals virtually, there is a certain provision of confidence and the knowledge their goals can indeed be realized. This visual representation of physicians from underrepresented demographics and the expanded formats have encouraged the call for more diversity in relatively homogenous fields, such as Orthopedic Surgery.

Another method of providing productive guidance to mentees is developing formal peer-support programs. Formal programs not only foster interest by sharing knowledge and teaching mentees about their passions, but it allows them to connect with mentors who have been identified as committed to the process. Mentors are connected directly with mentees. Mentees belonging to formal programs can feel more comfortable reaching out, asking questions, and building a relationship with a more experienced individual. Another nuance of the formal programs is the provision of expectations for both the mentor and the mentee to support the cultivation of a healthy, productive connection. This is different from the more organic approach to mentorship where expectations may not be clearly delineated.

Regardless of format, the most effective mentors bestow guidance toward professional opportunities and are truly invested in the success of the protégé. On the track to residency, professorship, or leadership, mentors should have the capacity to elevate. Sponsorship requires the additional step of advocacy. They carry the responsibility of guiding their pupil, promoting their positive contributions and attributes amongst colleagues, and truly advocating for the path forward at decision-making tables.

In **Fig. 1**, the general phases of mentorship are outlined, highlighting components of mentorship and sponsorship. Importantly, inclusive mentorship is identified and defined as mentoring across differences. Revisiting the question, *is mentorship available to everyone in the same quantity and the same quality*, chances are the responses to our inquiry will be mixed. The idea of inclusion is relatively new and many in positions of power are becoming more aware of the opportunities for creating an environment of belonging in our academic and clinical settings. Although there is rarely intent for disparate guidance and advocacy, those realities do exist and are borne out in the experiences, stories, and concerns of our diverse learners and faculty clinicians. Inclusive mentoring highlights the need of all mentors to be well-versed in the areas of stereotype threat, which is the contextual challenge in which individuals believe they are at risk of conforming to stereotypes about their social or demographic group. In addition, inclusive mentors recognize and circumvent issues

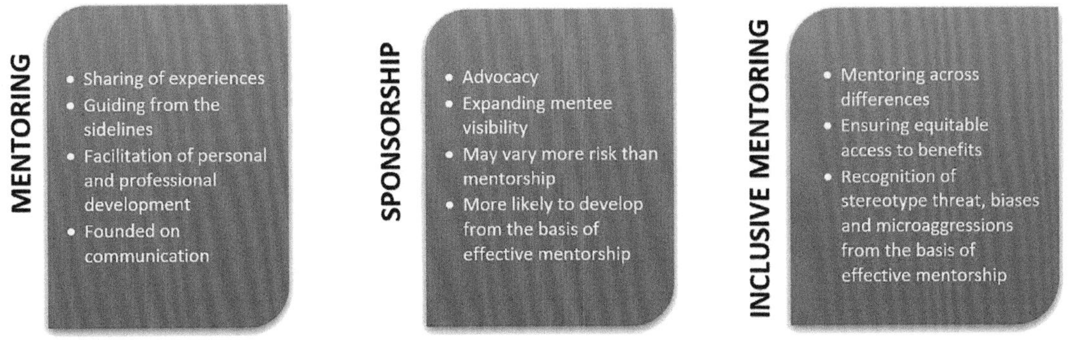
MENTORING
• Sharing of experiences
• Guiding from the sidelines
• Facilitation of personal and professional development
• Founded on communication
SPONSORSHIP
• Advocacy
• Expanding mentee visibility
• May vary more risk than mentorship
• More likely to develop from the basis of effective mentorship
INCLUSIVE MENTORING
• Mentoring across differences
• Ensuring equitable access to benefits
• Recognition of stereotype threat, biases and microaggressions from the basis of effective mentorship

Fig. 1. Phases of mentorship.

of bias and microaggressions. Lastly, inclusivity in this realm will ensure that the mentees have equitable access to the benefits of mentorship.

Indeed, it is human nature to intuitively search for mentors who share similar identity characteristics. However, for those who arguably could benefit the most from mentorship within orthopedic surgery, numbers of similar appearing mentors in academia are scarce. As a result, it is vital for physicians of all identity domains to avail themselves as mentors for members of diverse groups, with intent and inclusivity. Inclusive mentorship can elevate underrepresented populations in medicine and create intercultural relationships that can also benefit the relationships we have with our diversifying patient populations.

DEMOGRAPHICS IN ORTHOPEDIC SURGERY

Although Hand Surgery brings together teams from General Surgery, Orthopedic Surgery, and Plastic Surgery, Orthopedic Surgery is one of the most competitive medical specialties with a rapidly increasing number of applicants annually, yet stagnant progress in the area of diversity.[1] Thus, we will lean on the data from Orthopedic Surgery to show the case for inclusive mentorship. Despite the influx of applicants, Orthopedic Surgery continues to be one of the least diverse surgical specialties regarding sex and ethnicity.[2–4] Underrepresented minorities are defined by the Accreditation Council for Graduate Medical Education (ACGME) as African Americans, Latinos, and Native Americans/Alaskan natives. Within Orthopedic Surgery, Latinos/Hispanic, Black, American Indians, and Native Hawaiian/Pacific Islander physicians represent 2.2%, 1.9%, 0.4%, and 0.2%, respectively.[5] These statistics are drastically disproportionate to the overall US population of 18.7% Latinos/Hispanics, 14.2% African Americans/Black, 2.9% American Indian and 0.4% Pacific Islander[5] according to the 2020 census (**Fig. 2**).

Regarding sex, females currently represent 51% of all medical students. However, females only comprised 15.3% of residents and fellows, and 6.5% of American Academy of Orthopaedic Surgeons (AAOS) membership in 2019.[6,7] In fact, Acuña and colleagues analyzed trends in the annual percentage of women and determined it will take 217 years to obtain an equal proportion of men and women if Orthopedic Surgery continues growing at its current rate.[8–14]

Statisticians believe by 2045 current minorities in the United States will become the majority population, further solidifying the need for more diversity among health care professionals. In order to bridge this gap, inclusive mentorship and sponsorship are vital for the underrepresented demographics of Orthopedic Surgery. Mentors serve as a reminder of the achievable success. Mentors can also provide guidance with preparation and recruitment to residency programs and job placement. Furthermore, mentors can also serve as advocates to ensure their mentees receive appropriate opportunities. Finally, physicians in mentorship roles can assist when mentees experience common feelings of rejection, isolation, and sadness. Promoting inclusive mentorship and sponsorship is the next step to pushing the needle further within Orthopedic Surgery.

ACADEMIC PATHWAY DISPARITIES

To appreciate the necessity of inclusive mentorship, as well as the tools to incorporate it, it is prudent to acknowledge and understand the disparities that exist in an individual's pathway to surgery. From application to entry into a first job or leadership position, there are numerous obstacles and stacked odds that can be overcome by effective mentorship (guidance) and

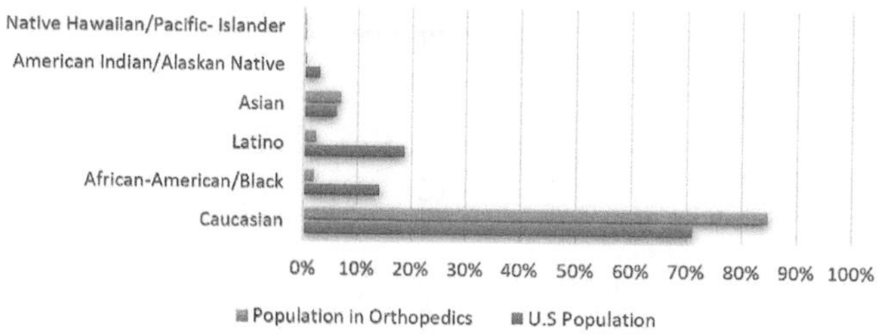

Fig. 2. Race and ethnicity in orthopedic surgery compared with 2020 US population.

sponsorship (advocacy) when done in an intentional manner.

Existing Disparities between Resident Applicants

With a startling match rate of 60% in 2022 (1,470 applicants for 875 positions), applicants strive for optimal preparation before entering the match process.[15] The highest United States Medical Licensing Examination (USMLE) scores and clerkship grades are encouraged. In addition, achieving Alpha Omega Alpha (AOA) status and an outstanding medical student performance evaluation (MSPE) can increase the odds of matching. There is an ongoing struggle to diversify applicants because of existing disparities seen with these residency application requirements.

Eugia and colleagues conducted a study in 2022 identifying commonalities in residents in surgery. They found residents in surgical specialties were less likely to come from disadvantaged backgrounds or have a family median income <$75,000. Students from disadvantaged backgrounds had a 50% decreased chance of entering the surgical field.[16–22] They also saw a family median income >$75,000 was associated with a higher NBME shelf exam score, increasing the ability to match into surgery. As NBME scores are positively correlated to USMLE scores, these findings expose the difficulty of matching into a surgical residency if an applicant stems from a disadvantaged background.[16,23]

High clerkship grades are required for an induction into Alpha Omega Alpha Honor Society. As a result, this inevitably affects the number of underrepresented minorities in AOA. The available literature already highlights the majority of Alpha Omega Alpha Honor medical society members are not Underrepresented Minority (URM) students.[24] The MSPE can also be disadvantageous for the URM student. The MSPE details a student's performance and sums up his/her tenure in one adjective (outstanding, excellent, very good, and good). Low and colleagues[25] showed independent of USMLE step scores, URM students had a lower chance of obtaining a description by the better superlatives.

The last step of the application process is the interview. In 2016, the average Orthopedic Surgery applicant applied to a median of 65 programs (range 21–88) and was offered a median of 15 interviews (range 15–25).[26] In-person interviews presented an additional financial burden on medical students, requiring many to take out additional loans.[26] Beginning in the era of COVID-19, virtual interviews presented new challenges of finding the perfect lighting, camera quality, and background. While removing the financial burden of an in-person interview, virtual interviews may still put some students at a disadvantage if they do not have the proper technology to make a great first impression with a residency program.

In summary, each aspect of the resident application process possesses risk for significant disparities between applicants of various demographics, especially those from a lower socioeconomic status (SES). Although the implementation of a holistic review of resident applicants has improved the number of underrepresented applications and matches, mentorship is one of the key differences between students who go matched and unmatched.[27]

The Impact of Limited Resources and Mentorship

Ulloa and colleagues reported a series of survey responses on the experience of African American and Latino surgeons. They found entry into medicine with a structured plan and appropriate mentorship versus an unstructured experience relying on self-discovery was strongly related to childhood SES.[28] Surgeons from a lower SES were completely unaware of whom or when to ask for assistance. Surgeons from a lower SES also noted unequal academic preparation before beginning medical school. Most importantly, the participants described significant struggles before finding mentorship. Many did not understand the nuance of critical decisions made along their career paths.

The Effects of Bias on a Resident's Psyche

Aryee and colleagues completed a study among 504 residents in multiple specialties examining the relationship between mentorship, feelings of isolation, and withdrawal. The authors found residents with greater access to mentorship displayed significantly decreased feelings of isolation.[29] Minority trainees experienced more challenges when executing orders and female trainees reported more instances of being labeled as staff with a lower training level (physician assistant, nurse, and lab tech) Ulloa and colleagues[28] surveyed African American and Latino surgeons who all described feeling isolated and/or working twice as hard to achieve equal recognition because of the color of their skin. Barnes and colleagues[30] found female surgical trainees experience more frequent, severe and stressful microagressions. These feelings can be difficult to process and can lead toward changing residencies or leaving medicine altogether. This can negatively affect the course of a resident's career, as well as the workflow of the hospital. Mentorship can teach residents how to combat challenges these obstacles.

Elevation into Leadership Positions

Mentorship and sponsorship are also imperative for elevation into positions of influence and power. In 2019, female medical students outnumbered men at 50.5% percent of the student population.[31] However, in that same year, according to an AAOS survey, 6.5% of 29,613 Orthopedic surgeons identified as women. Several residency programs have never hired a female resident.[32] In 2020, only 12.9% of women comprised residency and fellowship positions.[31] A study by Bi and colleagues[32] in 2022 found 27% of women are assistant program directors, 11% are program directors, 9% are division chiefs, 8% are vice chairs and only 3% are chairs among the 161 Orthopedic Surgery programs in the country. Having women and underrepresented minorities in leadership roles is essential to recruiting and retaining a diverse demographic of orthopedic surgeons. In addition, the Orthopaedic Diversity Leadership Consortium (ODLC) has identified the opportunities for empowerment of diversity leaders, including additional support, strategy development, education, and resources for the roles, that increase effectiveness in driving organizational change.

BARRIERS TO INCLUSIVE MENTORSHIP

Given the numerous proven areas of disparate opportunity, why is inclusive mentorship not promoted, discussed, or used? There are several barriers prohibiting inclusive mentorship to be widely accepted. These barriers center upon the current mindset of prospective mentors and potential obstacles to building a relationship with a mentee of a different background. We have separated these barriers into 6 categories: (1) traditional views of success, (2) lack of validation, (3) focus on rescue, (4) diminished value of achievements, (5) mixed goal agreement, and (6) mixed motivations (**Fig. 3**).

Traditional views of success are commonplace. In fact, as an example, Orthopedic Surgery has a very specific stereotype well known among medical students who announce they are interested in Orthopedic Surgery. These students will often get comments to solidify stereotypes that successful Orthopedic surgeons must have brawn and a certain pedigree. In addition, to be viewed as a successful applicant, many programs focus on number of publications, AOA status, and USMLE scores as surrogate markers. This mindset can deter potential mentors from forming meaningful relationships with mentees who do not meet these benchmarks or stereotypes and are from different backgrounds. This barrier is also encountered by faculty as well. Often, the templates used to guide promotion advancement (publications, society leadership, and awards) are used to determine whether a faculty surgeon is on track to be "successful." Interestingly, it is rare that our mentees or junior faculty are asked to define what success means to them. The medical community needs to expand the definition of success. For example, innovation, entrepreneurship, community service, investment in family and nonacademic personal achievement goals are also experiences that enhance skills as a physician and overall human being.

Lack of validation is another barrier to inclusive mentorship that is unfortunately experienced by many in Surgery, especially women and underrepresented minorities. Making excuses and invalidating one's experiences can be shown with common phrases like *"it's not them... it's you," "oh, that's just the way they are"*, *"that happens to everyone"*, or *"perhaps you're too sensitive."* Invalidation of experiences can negatively affect one's confidence and trust in authority figures who could have or currently serve as a mentor. Furthermore, imposter syndrome can be exacerbated when one's own trusted confidants and mentors minimize the magnitude of microaggressions. It is a well-known fact that minority students and physicians often suffer from imposter syndrome which has been correlated with depression

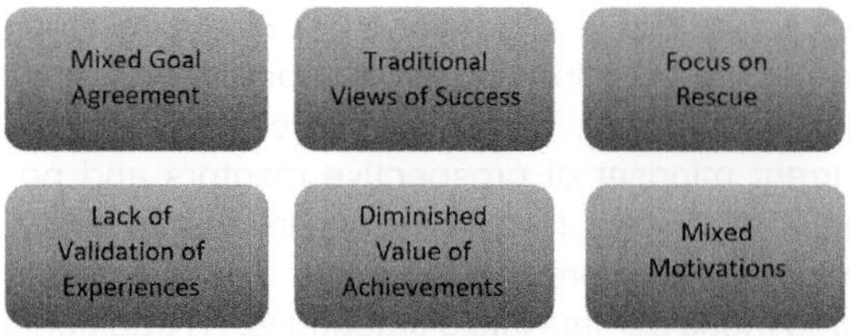

Fig. 3. Barriers to inclusive mentorship in orthopedic surgery.

and anxiety.[33,34] Lack of validation can further contribute to this phenomenon.

Another barrier is a presumptuous **focus on rescue** that many mentors lead with during their interactions. There is an assumption that all diverse mentees need to be pulled up to break through some sort of metaphorical glass ceiling. Although this may certainly be the case, it should not be assumed. There are many individuals who are at a place or position that brings them satisfaction and joy and they seek mentorship to optimize their success. By enforcing that the mentee "aim bigger" and "break barriers," we may apply undue stress on diverse individuals who are more interested in being provided equitable choice and opportunity in their current environment. Mentees generally have the grit, internal drive, and intelligence necessary to excel. They simply require an additional resource, including advisors with expertise and the ability to serve as an advocate.

Diminished value of achievements is a barrier that is often employed unknowingly. This involves pervasive "rising star" mentality and language. Even when an individual has gained several promotions, achieved his/her personal definition of success, and has excelled as a leader, they continue to be viewed as a "rising star," implying that they are still subordinate, or have incompletely arrived. This is a form of infantilizing that many diverse individuals are subject to when being addressed or discussed by majority counterparts. There is no clear consensus on when someone is no longer "potential" or "young" or "rising," but there should be some thoughtfulness when that terminology is used in describing minorities or women in professional settings. In surgical specialties, there is also no consensus based on using this language and it is unclear whether it is the individual's faculty appointment level, choice of social circles, level of society committee involvement, or the personal characteristics or identity that contribute to the infinite subordinate designation. It can be demeaning unintentionally, at which point the mentor or sponsor should be receptive to that feedback. It is the role of sponsors to advocate for their mentees in the form of speaking high and appropriate praises. If the mentee is frequently demoted or demeaned when discussed, it will be hard for colleagues to recognize their value and to treat them as equal peers.

The barriers to **mixed goal agreement** and **mixed motivation** refer to reasons for mentoring outside of altruism and connection. Mentorship roles, especially toward underrepresent populations, are at times sought after for academic promotion or professional/social media prestige instead of an actual invested interest in the individual. It can be damaging for the mentees to partner with mentors who are not truly serving their best interests. Eventually, the lack of true interest comes to light and can skew the view of our profession. Mentors should be equally committed to the mentorship process for learners and faculty of all backgrounds. The goals and expectations for the relationship will be individualized and that should be discussed toward the beginning of the interactions. There are indeed bidirectional benefits of the relationship, but without some substance behind the exchange, authenticity can be challenged.

NOW WHAT? APPROACHES TOWARD INCLUSIVE MENTORSHIP

We have outlined the evolution of mentorship, reviewed disparate experiences along the pathway, and identified real barriers to inclusive mentorship and sponsorship. The good news is that there are ways to mitigate these barriers and provide equitable mentorship experiences for all interested parties.

Embrace Differences

A solid first step is for us as a medical community to become comfortable working in a mentoring capacity with people from different backgrounds and communities. An ideology that has quickly gained traction over the past few decades is incorporating cultural humility and social determinants of health in medical education. After the US Department of Health and Human Services created the first review of ethnic and socioeconomic health care disparities, training on care for patients of various backgrounds began to become incorporated into the curriculum.[35] These curriculums familiarize future physicians with potential patient populations, as well as colleagues from diverse demographics who can serve as future mentors. We do not know what we do not know, so opening oneself to education on different cultures and identities is paramount for effective relationship formation.

Practice Humility

A healthy mentorship relationship is a bidirectional learning experience. Gone are the days when information is just passed from one older person to a younger person as a finite transaction. In fact, mentoring can occur at any chronological age, and position/power level does not always imply who is the provider or recipient of the mentoring. As such, all mentors must practice humility, as many mentees are already leaders and teachers, with amazing experiences to share. Our own intellectual and professional templates should not serve as the absolute benchmarks for success. Further, active listening should be employed with space made for the mentees to have a voice and influence. Mentors must also be able to recognize talent without fear of uplifting a mentee who has a nontraditional skillset. Furthermore, we must listen to the mentees' experience, allow them to feel validated, and create an avenue specific to that experience.

Empower

We described the "rescue" mentality as a barrier to true inclusive mentorship. The key to mitigation of this barrier is moving away from the "mentor as hero" narrative, and rather emphasizing the empowerment of the mentee. There is real value in encouraging mentees to take back control of situations or opportunities. Mentors can tap into their internal confidence and guide individuals through the complex political landscape that often plagues our clinical and academic environments. In addition, mentors can lead by equipping their learners or colleagues with the tools for in-the-moment action when microaggressions occur and, as a next step, can be active sponsors by advocating for increased respect and belonging in the workplace. This requires that mentors become better-versed in the frameworks used to optimize professionalism and navigate crucial conversations. When these tools are recognized and brought into play, we can shift from an escape-approach to a thrive-approach in our mentorship interactions.

Learn About Cognitive Biases

Our brain employs a multitude of cognitive biases that allow us to survive threats, perceived and real. Understanding the fine line between healthy survival use of biases, and the biases that can cause harm and loss of opportunity is critical for mentors and sponsors. For example, *anchoring bias* is the use of preexisting data as a reference point for all subsequent data. This can alter the decisions we make and influence the potential of others. In mentoring, this shows up when we compare individuals to an existing idea of what a surgeon—or leader—should look, sound, and behave. The antiquated prototype is the benchmark, and all other individuals are compared with that. *Confirmation bias*, on the contrary, causes us to seek out information and data that confirm our preexisting ideas to the point that we even ignore contrary information. This is frequently employed for diverse individuals at all levels of the surgical education and academic pathway. If a mentee is considered an "academic risk," or if a faculty peer mentee is labeled as "difficult," then any behavior that supports that narrative will be sought out and emphasized to confirm what was already believed, regardless of any performance, achievements, or skills that suggest the contrary. Of note, being academically risky or difficult are attributes disproportionately applied to diverse individuals. Another bias, known as the *framing bias*, is based on making decisions based on the way the information is presented, rather than based on the facts alone. This can impede effective sponsorship. How a mentee is discussed (what frames are used) impacts their pathway.

There are many more cognitive biases that we put in play, and they have been extensively studied. The more we educate ourselves about our cognitive biases, which we all have, and how they may manifest to the detriment of others, the better mentors will be at validating the experiences of diverse mentees and recognizing when the biases are entering our relationships.

Co-Create the Future

We have discussed the importance of breaking through traditional views of success in our mentorship relations. Another way to navigate through this area is to co-create the future with your mentee. Many surveys, focus groups, analyses, and exit interviews focus on the past, and sometimes the present: *what was, what is, what went well, and what is going wrong.* Rarely do we ask our mentees what an ideal future state would look like to them. By communicating with the mentees about their own views and visions of success, an inclusive future state of our profession can be created as a collaborative endeavor. With this approach, we will avoid some of the "hit and miss" iterations that can occur when majority populations decide what is best for others without any shared decision-making or dialogue in the process, apply the intervention, and then spend extensive time exploring why it did not work out. The co-creation process is not only more effective but confers levels of respect and belonging that excites both the mentor and mentee, thus strengthening the interaction.

Promote Resources for Mentorship

Many steps have already been taken to improve diversity, decrease biases, and foster mentorship. These resources, whether didactic courses or organizations, should be promoted by mentors and used as instruments to support success in the inclusive mentorship experience. For example, in Orthopedic Surgery, organizational pioneers who focus on these areas include the J. Robert Gladden foundation and the Ruth Jackson Orthopaedic Society. The J. Robert Gladden foundation named after the first African-American certified by the American Board of Orthopedic Surgery in 1949, was created in 1998. With the mission of increasing diversity in Orthopedic Surgery, mentorship is a key focus in JRGOS.[36] The creation of the annual JRGOS networking luncheon at the AAOS meeting, in-person and social media Q&A sessions, and financial aid provided for research and review courses has helped the 600 members.[36] Lastly, JRGOS members have been leaders in diversity, equity, and inclusion literature in Orthopedic Surgery, which continues altered the minds/culture of Orthopedic environments.

The Ruth Jackson Orthopedic Society, created in 1983, is an organization dedicated to uplifting women in Orthopedic Surgery. Ruth Jackson, a physician who experienced discrimination through her medical training and career, often working without pay, became the first female accepted into the American Academy of Orthopedic Surgery (AAOS).[37–39] A key focus of Ruth Jackson Orthopaedic Society (RJOS) is mentorship of a medical student, residents, and midcareer attendings. Mentorship includes mock interviews, grant writing tips, CV and cover letter templates, mock and exams for the American Board of Orthopaedic Surgeons (ABOS) examination.[37] RJOS also provides scholarships and traveling fellowships.[37]

Black Women Orthopaedic Surgeons (BWOS) and American Association of Latino Orthopaedic Surgeons (AALOS) are additional organizations that have blossomed within the last several years. The Perry Initiative and Nth Dimensions are pioneering pipeline programs for premedical and medical students that provide exposure and mentorship for students passionate about Orthopedic Surgery. The presence of these organizations is imperative to provide a voice for groups within Orthopedic Surgery that are small in number.

As we move into the leadership pathways, the ODLC has carved out a critical space for resources and support of diversity, equity, and inclusion leaders across the United States and internationally. Through formal courses, strategy sessions, networking events, and monthly "Transformation Talks," Diversity, Equity, and Inclusion (DEI) leaders, most of whom are also practicing surgeons, come together to share best practices, understand organizational dynamics, and learn strategic frameworks on how to create effective, sustainable change across all dimensions of diversity in a multitude of environments. This organization has been very effective for faculty and learners who serve in diversity-focused leadership roles that are intrinsically challenging yet gratifying. Many mentor-mentee leadership relationships have been established through the power of this network.

SUMMARY

Mentorship and sponsorship are two vital components to professional and personal success and have become a mainstay in many academic and clinical environments. Without a doubt, there are still several barriers prohibiting inclusive mentorship from being widely understood and employed. There is much opportunity in our surgical fields to bridge gaps, subtle and macro in size, and bring respect, belonging, and empathy to our environments. The disparities begin earlier than is recognized and occur through multiple parts of one's journey.

Fortunately, there are solution-based approaches that can be taken to mitigate these obstacles and form healthy, inclusive mentoring relationships. We can engage with the pioneering organizations that have leaned into the complex work of diversity, equity, and inclusion for additional support, insight, and resources. Our mentees deserve the best guidance and advocacy we can provide, which will significantly benefit the patients and communities we are gratefully obligated to serve.

CLINICS CARE POINTS

Pearls

- Surgeons from a lower socioeconomic status benefit from more guidance through mentorship—often unaware of whom or when to ask for assistance and struggling significantly on the premedical track.[28]

- Students from disadvantaged backgrounds had a 50% decreased chance of entering the surgical field. They are more likely to have lower National Board of Medical Examiners (NBME) shelf scores, USMLE scores, and Alpha Omega Alpha status.[15,23]
- Female surgical trainees experience more frequent, severe and stressful microagressions.[30]
- There are several mentorship organizations focusing on inclusive mentorship of medical student, residents, and midcareer attendings through one or one relationships, formal courses, strategy sessions, and networking events.[36,37]

Pitfalls

- Documented barriers to effective mentorship include mismatched expectations between mentor and mentee, lack of available mentors, lack of time/compensation for mentors, and geographic separation between mentor and mentee.[40]
- Many physicians in the workplace do not feel their institution supports mentorship in the workplace.[40]
- Without institutional support, the workplace environment does not demand inclusion and responsibility of promoting this environment falls on individuals, not the workplace.[40]

DISCLOSURE

Consultant for Johnson & Johnson DePuy Synthes. Founder of the Orthopedic Diversity Leadership Consortium. Sponsored by Stryker, Total Joint Orthopedics, Tru-Color, and Johnson & Johnson DePuy Synthes.

REFERENCES

1. Schrock JB, Kraeutler MJ, Dayton MR, et al. A comparison of matched and unmatched orthopaedic surgery residency applicants from 2006 to 2014: data from the national resident matching program. J Bone Joint Surg Am 2017;99(1):e1.
2. Day CS, Lage DE, Ahn CS. Diversity based on race, ethnicity, and sex between academic orthopaedic surgery and other specialties: a comparative study. J Bone Joint Surg Am 2010;92(13):2328–35.
3. Poon S, Kiridly D, Mutawakkil M, et al. Current trends in sex, race, and ethnic diversity in orthopaedic surgery residency. J Am Acad Orthop Surg 2019;27(16):e725–33.
4. Poon SC, Nellans K, Gorroochurn P, et al. Race, but not gender, is associated with admissions into orthopaedic residency programs. Clin Orthop Relat Res 2020;480(8):1441–9.
5. McDonald TC, Drake LC, Replogle WH, et al. Barriers to increasing diversity in orthopaedics: the residency program perspective. JB JS Open Access 2020;5(2).
6. Chambers CC, Ihnow SB, Monroe EJ, et al. Women in orthopaedic surgery: population trends in trainees and practicing surgeons. J Bone Joint Surg Am 2018;100(17):e116.
7. Van Heest A. Gender diversity in orthopedic surgery: we all know it's lacking, but why? Iowa Orthop J 2020;40(1):1–4.
8. Acuna AJ, Sato EH, Jella TK, et al. How long will it take to reach gender parity in orthopaedic surgery in the united states? An analysis of the national provider identifier Registry. Clin Orthop Relat Res 2021;479(6):1179–89.
9. Dykes DC, White AA 3rd. Getting to equal: strategies to understand and eliminate general and orthopaedic health care disparities. Clin Orthop Relat Res 2009;467(10):2598–605.
10. Betancourt JR, Carrillo JE, Green AR. Hypertension in multicultural and minority populations: linking communication to compliance. Curr Hypertens Rep 1999;1(6):482–8.
11. Saha S, Freeman M, Toure J, et al. Racial and ethnic disparities in the VA health care system: a systematic review. J Gen Intern Med 2008;23(5):654–71.
12. Sedlis SP, Fisher VJ, Tice D, et al. Racial differences in performance of invasive cardiac procedures in a Department of Veterans Affairs Medical Center. J Clin Epidemiol 1997;50(8):899–901.
13. Hannan EL, van Ryn M, Burke J, et al. Access to coronary artery bypass surgery by race/ethnicity and gender among patients who are appropriate for surgery. Med Care 1999;37(1):68–77.
14. Hoenig H, Rubenstein L, Kahn K. Rehabilitation after hip fracture–equal opportunity for all? Arch Phys Med Rehabil 1996;77(1):58–63.
15. The Match NRMP. Main Residency Match Data and Reports, Available at: https://www.nrmp.org/match-data-analytics/residency-data-reports/.
16. Eguia E, Kolachina S, Miller E, et al. Medical students from socioeconomically disadvantaged backgrounds are less likely to match into surgery. World J Surg 2022;46(6):1261–7.
17. Steel N, Clark A, Lang IA, et al. Racial disparities in receipt of hip and knee joint replacements are not explained by need: the Health and Retirement Study 1998-2004. J Gerontol A Biol Sci Med Sci 2008;63(6):629–34.
18. Schairer WW, Nwachukwu BU, Warren RF, et al. Operative fixation for clavicle fractures-socioeconomic differences persist despite overall population increases in utilization. J Orthop Trauma 2017;31(6):e167–72.

19. Zelle BA, Morton-Gonzaba NA, Adcock CF, et al. Health care disparities among orthopedic trauma patients in the USA: socio-demographic factors influence the management of calcaneus fractures. J Orthop Surg Res 2019;14(1):359.
20. Saha S, Komaromy M, Koepsell TD, et al. Patient-physician racial concordance and the perceived quality and use of health care. Arch Intern Med 1999;159(9):997–1004.
21. Shen MJ, Peterson EB, Costas-Muniz R, et al. The effects of race and racial concordance on patient-physician communication: a systematic review of the literature. J Racial Ethn Health Disparities 2018;5(1):117–40.
22. Menendez ME, van Hoorn BT, Mackert M, et al. Patients with limited health literacy ask fewer questions during office visits with hand surgeons. Clin Orthop Relat Res 2017;475(5):1291–7.
23. Raborn LN, Janis JE. Current views on the new united states medical licensing examination step 1 pass/fail format: a review of the literature. J Surg Res 2022;274:31–45.
24. Williams M, Kim EJ, Pappas K, et al. The impact of United States Medical Licensing Exam (USMLE) step 1 cutoff scores on recruitment of underrepresented minorities in medicine: a retrospective cross-sectional study. Health Sci Rep 2020;3(2):e2161.
25. Low D, Pollack SW, Liao ZC, et al. Racial/ethnic disparities in clinical grading in medical school. Teach Learn Med 2019;31(5):487–96.
26. Fogel HA, Finkler ES, Wu K, et al. The economic burden of orthopedic surgery residency interviews on applicants. Iowa Orthop J 2016;36:26–30.
27. Sungar WG, Angerhofer C, McCormick T, et al. Implementation of holistic review into emergency medicine residency application screening to improve recruitment of underrepresented in medicine applicants. AEM Educ Train 2021;5(Suppl 1):S10–8.
28. Ulloa JG, Viramontes O, Ryan G, et al. Perceptual and structural facilitators and barriers to becoming a surgeon: a qualitative study of african american and latino surgeons. Acad Med 2018;93(9):1326–34.
29. Aryee JNA, Bolarinwa SA, Montgomery SR Jr, et al. Race, gender, and residency: a survey of trainee experience. J Natl Med Assoc 2021;113(2):199–207.
30. Barnes KL, McGuire L, Dunivan G, et al. Gender bias experiences of female surgical trainees. J Surg Educ 2019;76(6):e1–14.
31. Dib AG, Lowenstein NA, LaPorte DM, et al. The pioneering women of orthopaedic surgery: a historical review. J Bone Joint Surg Am 2022.
32. Bi AS, Fisher ND, Bletnitsky N, et al. Representation of women in academic orthopaedic leadership: where are we now? Clin Orthop Relat Res 2022;480(1):45–56.
33. Campbell KM, Tumin D, Infante Linares JL. The need for better studies of impostor syndrome in underrepresented minority faculty. Acad Med 2021;96(5):617.
34. Gottlieb M, Chung A, Battaglioli N, et al. Impostor syndrome among physicians and physicians in training: A scoping review. Med Educ 2020;54(2):116–24.
35. Butler PD, Swift M, Kothari S, et al. Integrating cultural competency and humility training into clinical clerkships: surgery as a model. J Surg Educ 2011;68(3):222–30.
36. Brooks JT, Taylor E, Peterson D, et al. The J. Robert gladden orthopaedic society: past, present, and future. J Am Acad Orthop Surg 2022;30(8):344–9.
37. Samora JB, Russo C, LaPorte D. Ruth jackson orthopaedic society: promoting women in orthopaedics. J Am Acad Orthop Surg 2022;30(8):364–8.
38. Cannada LK, O'Connor MI. Equity360: gender, race, and ethnicity-harassment in orthopaedics and #SpeakUpOrtho. Clin Orthop Relat Res 2021;479(8):1674–6.
39. Whicker E, Williams C, Kirchner G, et al. What proportion of women orthopaedic surgeons report having been sexually harassed during residency training? A survey study. Clin Orthop Relat Res 2020;478(11):2598–606.
40. Bonifacino E, Ufomata EO, Farkas AH, et al. Mentorship of underrepresented physicians and trainees in academic medicine: a systematic review. J Gen Intern Med 2021;36(4):1023–34.

Women in Hand Surgery
Leadership and Legacy

Wendy Chen, MD, MS[a,*], Allyne Topaz, MD[b]

KEYWORDS

• Diversity • Pregnancy • Female • Women • Hand surgery • Leadership • History • Advocacy

KEY POINTS

- Women have struggled for their place in the surgical discipline for thousands of years. Today, women in medicine, surgery, and Hand Surgery are increasing, but the history of this journey has not been recorded.
- Entrée to Hand Surgery includes effective mentorship, sponsorship, equitable training opportunities, research, funding, and engagement in national and international societies.
- Female Hand surgeons have made paradigm-changing contributions to the field of Hand Surgery.
- All hand surgeons should know the history of our specialty, its culture, and how to become active allies for contributing to our shared community.

No woman studying medicine today will ever know how much it has cost the individuals personally concerned in bringing about these changes; how eagerly they have watched new developments and mourned each defeat and rejoiced with each success. For with them it meant much more than success or failure for the individual, it meant the failure or success of a grand cause.

—1899, Dr Marie Mergler, Dean of Woman's Hospital Medical College[1]

HISTORICAL BACKGROUND

The ideal surgeon should have the eye of an eagle, the heart of a lion, and the hands of a woman.

—Fifteenth century English proverb[2]

The history of surgery dates as far as 5000 years,[3] with hand fractures described as early as 300 BC, by Hippocrates. The history of women in surgery dates to 3500 BCE, with historical roles in Egypt, Italy, and Greece.[4–6] The Middle Ages saw women expressly banned from medicine and even burned as witches. Nevertheless, for hundreds of years, women persisted (**Fig. 1**), clandestinely, in monasteries; through midwifery and gynecology; and, in the 1700 to 1800s, presenting themselves as men to pursue medical education (**Fig. 2**).

Although not a hand surgeon, as the first American female board-certified orthopedic surgeon, Dr Ruth Jackson (**Fig. 3**) was a pioneer and founder of the eponymous orthopedic society for women. Graduating from Baylor in 1928, she was one of four women in a class of more than 100. Despite great deterrence, she pursued orthopedic surgery residency, only to begin her practice in Dallas, TX, during the Great Depression, earning $3/h from the Work Projects Administration as part of the New Deal.

When the American Academy of Orthopaedic Surgery (AAOS) was founded, all male orthopedic surgeons were grandfathered into membership, but Dr Jackson, then Chief of Orthopedics at Parkland Hospital, was required to first pass the American Board of Orthopaedic Surgery (ABOS) examination, which she did in 1937. Some decades later, Dr Marybeth Ezaki would rotate through Parkland Hospital as a medical student,

[a] University of Texas at Houston McGovern Medical School, 6410 Fannin Street, Suite 1400, Houston, TX 77030, USA; [b] Plastic Surgery, The University of Texas Medical Branch, 301 University Boulevard, Galveston, TX 77555-0724, USA
* Corresponding author.
E-mail address: wendy.chen@uth.tmc.edu

Hand Clin 39 (2023) 53–64
https://doi.org/10.1016/j.hcl.2022.08.024
0749-0712/23/Published by Elsevier Inc.

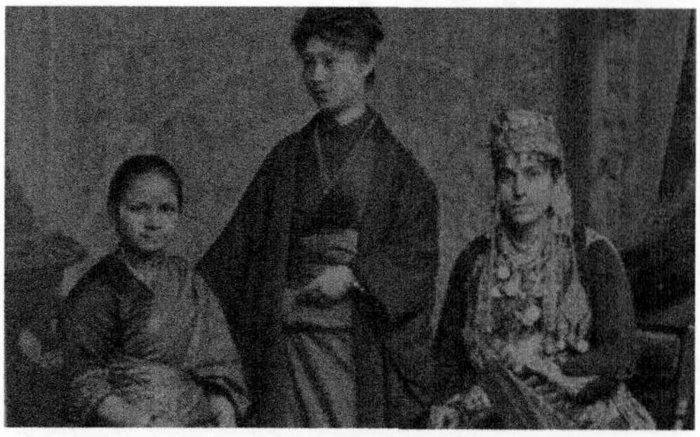

Fig. 1. The first female physicians from India, Japan, and Syria. (*Left to right*) Anandibal Joshi (India); Keiko Okami (Japan); Sabat Islambouli (Syria). They were students at the Women's Medical College of Pennsylvania in 1885, and the first women from their respective countries to matriculate in Western medicine. (Anandibai Joshee, Kei Okami, and Tabat M. Islambool, Author unknown via Wikimedia Commons / Public Domain.)

and, among other accomplishments, become the first female director of the ABOS.[7]

In 1948, Dr Alma Dea Morani (**Fig. 4**) became the first female surgeon admitted to the American Society of Plastic and Reconstructive Surgeons (ASPS). Born in New York City in 1907, her father was an acclaimed sculptor and believed medicine was too difficult a career for women. And indeed, there were challenges—as the only female physician, her living quarters were relegated to nursing quarters. After earning board certification in general surgery, it took six applications to Plastic Surgery before Dr Barrett Brown accepted her as a trainee (St Louis, 1946). Yet, she was only permitted to observe during the week. Solely on Saturdays, when the male residents had their day off, was she permitted to scrub and assist with surgery.

Dr Morani is responsible for establishing Philadelphia's first Hand Surgery Clinic (1958) and cofounding the Robert H. Ivy Society of Plastic Surgery. She advocated for women throughout her life, through the American Medical Women's Association and as president of the Medical Women's International Association.[8]

Organized Hand Surgery and Birth of Hand Societies

What we know now as organized, modern Hand Surgery as a specialty originated in the Second World War, with Dr Sterling Bunnell, who was tasked to lead the "crippled hand" service for the Medical Corps of the Army.[9] Through his work developing Hand Centers and training surgeons, The American Society for Surgery of the Hand (ASSH) was founded in Chicago at the January 1946 annual meeting of the AAOS, at the Blackstone Hotel.

But the ASSH was exclusive. "For many years, the forward rows in the audience were cordoned off with a velvet rope, and nonmembers ventured into their area at their peril."[10] Because of its stringent annual admission quota of ten new members, junior hand surgeons seeking to exchange knowledge began to organize in other ways. In 1970, the American Association for Hand Surgery (AAHS) was founded, "at an airport hotel near Chicago…to eliminate the elitist attitude for membership."[11]

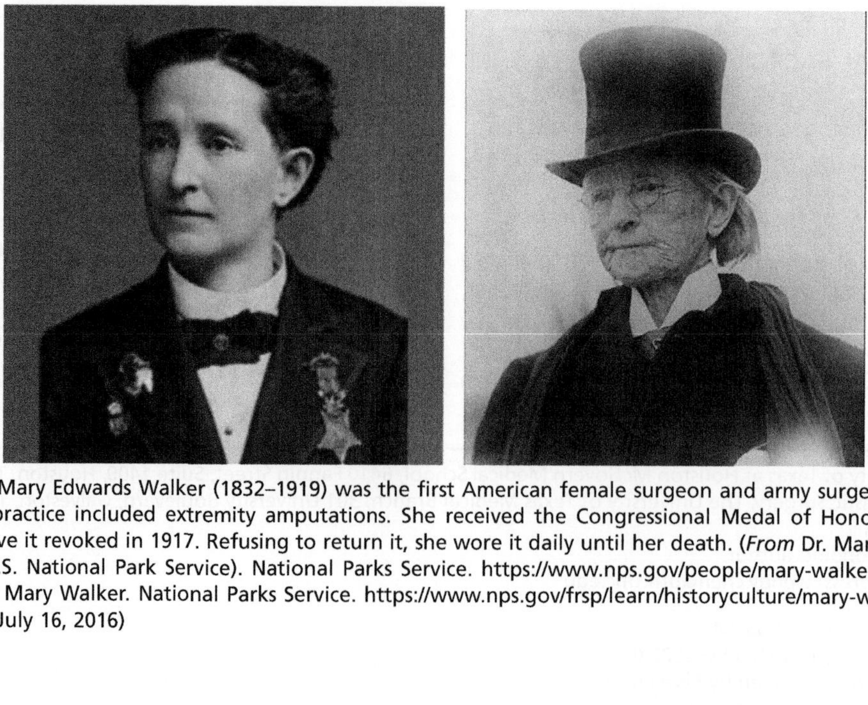

Fig. 2. Dr Mary Edwards Walker (1832–1919) was the first American female surgeon and army surgeon, whose scope of practice included extremity amputations. She received the Congressional Medal of Honor in 1865, only to have it revoked in 1917. Refusing to return it, she wore it daily until her death. (*From* Dr. Mary Edwards Walker (U.S. National Park Service). National Parks Service. https://www.nps.gov/people/mary-walker.htm; and Lavelle M. Mary Walker. National Parks Service. https://www.nps.gov/frsp/learn/historyculture/mary-walker.htm. Published July 16, 2016)

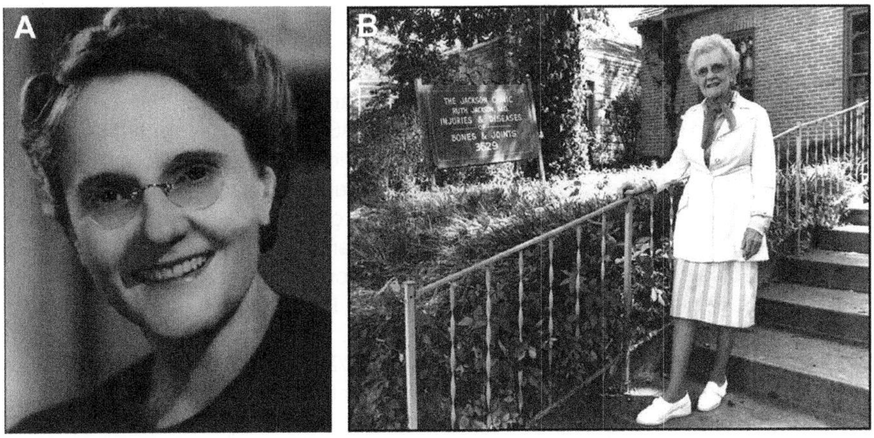

Fig. 3. (*A*) Dr Ruth Jackson. (*B*) On the right, age 84, outside of her clinic at Baylor University Medical Center in 1986. ([*A*]*Courtesy of* Ruth Jackson Orthopaedic Society, Schaumburg, IL; with permission.)

The Beginnings of Female Surgeons in Hand Societies

Females are aware of our inherent difficulties; knowing the barriers and help[ing] to speak to that... Unless you have female representation... the institutional barriers will persist - Dr. Ann Van Heest

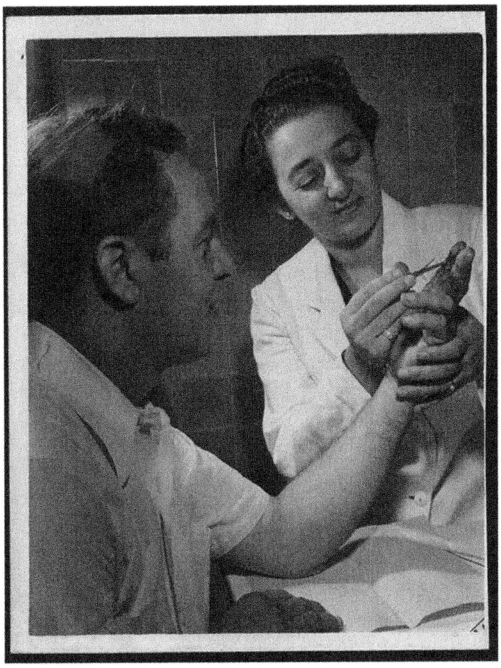

Fig. 4. Dr Alma Dea Morani repairs the damaged fingers of a patient in the hand clinic, undated. (https://drexel.edu/legacy-center/the-collections/exhibits/professors-from-the-past/alma-dea-morani/Legacy Center Archives, Drexel University College of Medicine, Philadelphia.)

*It has been a challenge to be president of these societies; there have been only one or no women in leadership of these societies...It's not important that it be 50% women, but it is important they be present because it makes something different, you can address the whole community and it brings diversity..." We [women] have a tendency to think we aren't good enough- we need to believe in ourselves and not wait for someone to call on us to promote us... no one at the table will give you a piece of the cake- you have to say it's for you" -Dr. Eva-Maria Baur**

*—*Dr Baur has served as President of the German Hand Surgery Society, President of International Wrist Arthroscopy Society, and will serve as President of the National Hand Society.*

For the first 50 years of ASSH history very little was written about female hand surgeons.[10] Although few in number, their contributions to science and leadership have been profound.

In 1984, Dr Julia Terzis was the first female surgeon to win the Emanuel B. Kaplan Award for "anatomic excellence in surgery of the hand" for her work describing the organization of the median nerve. Dr Susan E. Mackinnon followed in 1985, for her work on the lateral antebrachial cutaneous nerve and superficial sensory branch of the radial nerve.

The first time a female surgeon won an ASSH research grant was in 1986, and there were multiple: Dr Mackinnon ("The Nerve Allograft Response- An Immunologic Study with Cyclosporin A"), Dr Sharon A. Clark ("The Reorganization of the Somatosensory Cortex Following Ulnar Island Pedicle Flap to the Face in an Animal Model"), and Dr Terzis ("Effects of Pulsed

Electromagnetic Field on Nerve Regeneration"). Dr Amy Ladd was the first female surgeon to win the Sterling Bunnell Traveling Fellowship in Hand Surgery (2000).

The only female surgeon to serve in leadership in these first fifty years was Dr Elizabeth A. Ouellette, first on the Council in 1993, with the sponsorship of Dr Robert Hotchkiss, and then, as Co-Chair of the Business of Hand Surgery Committee, Vice President of the Kiros Society for Hand Research, Inc, and President of the Ruth Jackson Orthopaedic Society. She was also the Hand surgeon for Miami Heat, the Dolphins, the Panthers, and multiple universities, while continuing basic science research.

From 1995 to 2002, Dr Marybeth Ezaki (**Fig. 5**) and Dr Joan Wright were the only two women to serve on the council, and in 2002, as an American woman of Polish and Japanese descent, Dr Ezaki became the first female to serve as president of the ASSH in its 56-year history. She remains the only woman to have served in this role and recalls being "pushed through a door that was opened for her."[12] (In 2022, Dr Jennifer Wolf became the second.)

In the 2000s, more women began to gain admission to the Council. Before election to the Council, Dr Kay Kirkpatrick had already led the Georgia Orthopaedic Society and spent five years legislating as a Georgia State Senator. Her focus was on practice management and insurance issues affecting hand surgeons.

Encouraged by the few female role models before her, Dr Julie Katarincic (Mayo Clinic Hand Surgery Fellowship, Class of 1995) wanted to encourage others like her to get involved. She has worked with multiple committees within the society to improve diversity, including the Nominations Committee, and now heads the Outreach Division and advocates for sustainable education outreach and volunteering through Touching Hands. She is a professor at Albert Medical School at Brown University.

Dr Anne Miller (Tufts Hand Surgery Fellowship, Class of 1989) joined the board of the American Foundation of Surgery of the Hand early on and rose to leadership by serving on the board, including as President for four years. She helped create the bylaws and the criteria for the nominating committee and lead the Future in Hand Capital Campaign. In the 1980s, navigating Orthopedic and Hand Surgery was rife with obstacles–accessing residency, fellowship, family planning, and starting practice. Dr Miller is in private practice and volunteers with the Healing the Children Group, who honored her for her work with children with congenital hand differences. She has always wanted to have a voice and to promote fairness in society leadership. She currently serves as the RVS Update Committee for the American Medical Association advisor for Hand Surgery, and as chair of the ASSH Coding Committee.

Dr Michelle Carlson (Hospital for Special Surgery Hand Surgery Fellowship, Class of 1993) served on the ASSH Board for six years and as treasurer from 2014 to 2017, and is cited as a role model by many women. Throughout her career, Dr Carlson has won several prestigious awards, including the Ruth Jackson Orthopaedic Society/Zimmer Research Grant, the Lewis Clark Wagner Research Award, the T. Campbell Thompson Prize, and the Glasgow Memorial Achievement Citation. Dr Carlson is the director and founder of the Children and Adolescent Hand and Arm Center, the official second opinion physician for the NBA, as well as consultant hand surgeon for several professional sports teams.

Member-at-large on Council, Dr Dawn Laporte (Curtis National Hand Center Hand Surgery Fellowship, Class of 2001) has mentored innumerable trainees, particularly through her work with the resident education committee, resident educator workshop, and resident and fellow review courses. She is a Section Editor for the Journal of Hand Surgery, residency program director at Johns Hopkins University, and was Vice Chair for the ACGME Orthopaedic Surgery Residency Review Committee.

In 2022, Dr Jennifer Wolf (Mayo Clinic Hand Surgery Fellowship, Class of 2003) became the second female president of the ASSH. A full professor, she directs the Hand Surgery fellowship at the University of Chicago and serves as Vice Chair for faculty mentoring and diversity. Throughout her career, she was often the only woman in the room—the only female Hand Surgery fellow, the only female faculty member. Since being recruited to Chicago, she has hired seven women onto faculty and makes a point to invest in her juniors.

American Association for Hand Surgery

Since its inception, female hand therapists have had a much more prominent position, visibility, and leadership in AAHS than female hand surgeons.[11] Their story is no less important, but beyond the scope of this article. In 1978, Dr Mary H. McGrath was the first woman to win the resident essay award; two years later, Elizabeth J. Hall (renowned now as Dr Hall-Findlay) was the second female awardee, in third place. Dr McGrath, who would later become the first female president of the ASPS, started her years-long tenure heading the education committee (1983–

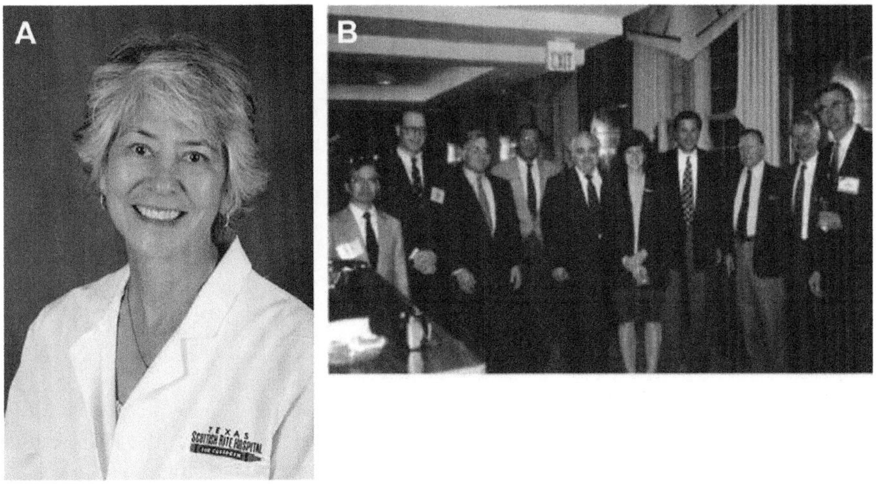

Fig. 5. (*A*) Dr Marybeth Ezaki. (B) Founder's meeting of Congenital Hand Anomalies Study Group (CHASG). ([*A*] *Courtesy of* Marybeth Ezaki, MD; [*B*] *From* Foucher G. Ten years CHASG, a combination of science and friendship. Handchir Mikrochir Plast Chir. 2004;36(2-3):189-190. https://doi.org/10.1055/s-2004-817886; with permission.)

1987), and Jean Kiefer began editing the newsletter committee (1983). Kristin Steuber was the first woman to head the Resident Essay Committee (1986) and the first woman to head the Nominating Committee (1988). Dr Stueber later became Chief of Plastic Surgery at Temple University Hospital, the second woman to hold such chairmanship in the country.[13]

It was not until 2005, 35 years after the founding of AAHS, that Susan E. Mackinnon (**Fig. 6**) became the first woman to serve as president, and she remains singular in that accomplishment. Her scientific contributions are separately discussed. When she was chosen, "Christine Novak PT, PhD was a natural choice as the first therapist/Program Chair." With the intention of increasing the visibility of the Association and advancing the science of hand care beyond Hand Surgery, Dr Mackinnon conceived and initiated *HAND* as the Association's Journal. Since the first issue in 2007, *HAND* has grown to six issues a year and is indexed in Medline.[14] Furthermore, during her leadership, the inaugural Alan Freeland Award was established to honor his relentless and selfless dedication to promoting the best Hand Surgery and hand therapy care around the world.

Hand Surgery Fellowships

Don't come if you're looking for a husband"

You're coming because [Dr. X] wants you... I don't believe women belong in Orthopaedics...

I will never take a woman. Over my dead body...

If you get pregnant, have a complication and are out for more than four weeks- I will fire you
—Various Faculty and Chairmen, 1980s

How should we contact you when you're out [on maternity leave]call the beauty shop?
—Private Practice, Midwest, 1980s

Residency Interviewer: "Won't it be difficult to work if you have your menses?"

Female Applicant (Future Hand Surgeon): "I have it right now..."

-Fellowship Interview, 1990s.
—Quotes from female Hand surgeons interviewed for this article.

The accessibility of Hand Surgery fellowships to women has evolved over the decades. Once a rarity, female surgeons now represent one-quarter of Hand Surgery fellowship graduates.[15]

Before efforts to standardize Hand Surgery fellowships, access to training was gated, and one could practice Hand Surgery without subspecialty training. A third-party algorithm now services the current "match" system, whereas historically, a phone call with an offer would be extended, with an assigned grace period (often quoted at 24 hours) to accept the position. The CAQ examination was subsequently developed as a certification to gain admission to ASSH membership, the first examination being administered in 1989. It is now known as the Subspecialty Certificate in Surgery of the Hand (SCC). SSC was open to

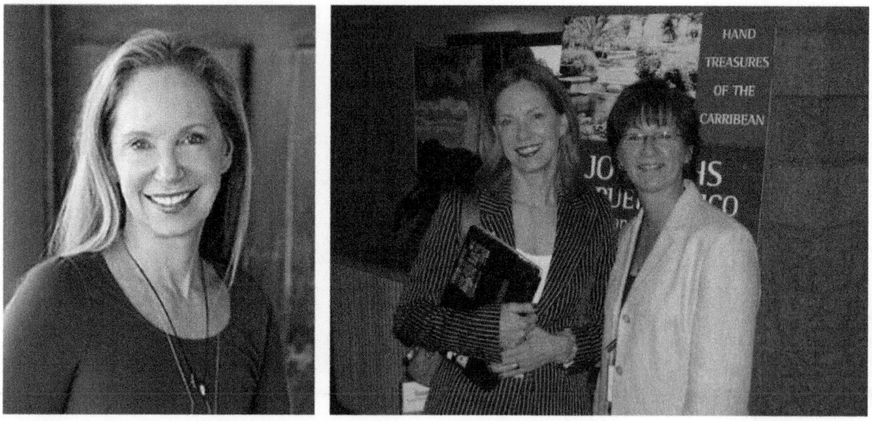

Fig. 6. Dr Susan Mackinnon, right, with Program Chair Christine Novak, PT, PhD, at the 2006 Annual Meeting. (*Courtesy of* Susan Mackinnon, MD and Christine Novak, PT, PhD.)

Diplomats of the 3 boards- General Surgery, Plastic Surgery, and Orthopaedic Surgery, with a trilateral committee overseeing the content, review, and standardized passing score. The first woman on the board of the ABOS, Dr Ezaki chaired this committee while on the ABOS, before serving as the director of the ABOS, Chair of the Maintenance of Certification (MOC) committee, and has made major contributions to the current American Hand Surgery fellowship structure and board examination process. Dr Ezaki was recently honored as a Pioneer in Hand Surgery by the IFSSH in 2022.

In the 1980s, female Hand Surgery fellows were scarce. So much so, multiple facilities still required them to wear the traditional scrub dress reserved for women (**Fig. 7**). Dr Michelle James and Dr Jeanne DelSignore (first female Hand Surgery fellows, Indiana Hand Center, 1988) remember the lack of changing facilities for female physicians. A broom closet was converted into a locker space for the two women, eventually guarded by a specialty lock designed to limit immediate entrance from the hallway. Similarly, Dr Ann Miller (Tufts, 1989) recounts the only entry to the dictation room required passage through the male locker room.

Applying to Hand Surgery fellowship in the 1990s, Dr Lattanza (Chair of Orthopaedics, Yale University, current; St. Lukes Roosevelt, 1999) was told letters of recommendation were not written for women. Even so, multiple surgeons who trained during this era agreed that so long as you did the work, you were regarded in a gender-neutral fashion. In the military, Dr Charlotte E. Alexander (Captain, Medical Corps, US Navy; Navy Sterling-Bunnell Hand Surgery Fellowship, 1983) felt highly supported and encouraged during her fellowship years.

In recent years, we have started to see instances of all-female fellowship classes, maternity leave policies, and lactation rooms.

Formation of Interest Groups

In 1983, the Ruth Jackson Orthopaedic Society was established "to promote professional development of and for women in orthopedics throughout all stages of their career." The founding

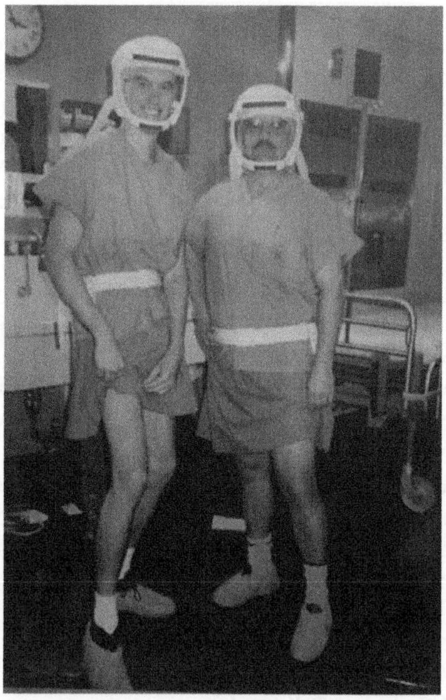

Fig. 7. Orthopaedic Surgery attending surgeon and resident wore "scrub dresses" in a during Halloween at the hospital. This "scrub dress" was common attire for female surgeons in the Northeast United States during the 1970s-1980s. (*Courtesy of* Eric Sides, MD, Danny Gurba, MD, and Liza Lattanza, MD, FAOA, FAAOS.)

members included Dr Jackson herself, Dr Liebe S. Diamond, and four other female Orthopedic surgeons.

Multiple female Hand surgeons have served as President of this society, including Dr Mary Lynn Newport (1998), Dr Ouellette (2007), Dr Ann Van Heest (2009), Dr Michelle James (2012), Dr Lisa Lattanza (2017), and Dr Dawn LaPorte (2020). In 2019, the society implemented a new award ("He For She") to recognize a male Orthopedic surgeon who serves as a strong mentor and sponsor for women in orthopedics, supporting and empowering females at all stages of their careers to achieve their professional goals.[16]

At the 2012 ASSH meeting, Drs Michelle Carlson, Dawn Laporte, Jennifer Wolf, Julie Katarincic, and Ann Van Heest decided there was a need for networking among the few existing female Hand surgeons, and the *Women in Hand Surgery (WISH)* group was born in a hallway in Chicago. After that first unofficial gathering, the ASSH has since adopted and funded the group.

Last, most recently, social media (Instagram, Facebook) has also served as a vehicle for female Hand surgeons of various training backgrounds to coalesce.

Mentorship

> *Mentors give advice, listen to you whine and celebrate your wins, help with career decisions, and a sponsor is someone who gives you a hand and pulls you forward. Marybeth [Ezaki] was doing this behind the scenes for me without me even knowing...*
>
> *—Dr. Lisa Lattanza*

With so few women, the history of mentorship of female hand surgeons has largely relied on male allies, from accessing residency training, to navigating early practice and research, to leadership positions.

In 2009, while bonding over how to succeed in male-dominated fields, *the Perry Initiative* (named after Dr Jaquelin Perry) was conceived by Dr Jennie Buckley, PhD, a biomechanical engineer at the University of California at San Francisco (UCSF) and Dr Lisa Lattanza. This nonprofit began as a weekend program for 18 girls, and has since grown to a national outreach program with more than 14,000 young women participating in the program since its inception. In 2021, 60 women who matched into orthopedics had been graduates of the Perry Program. Students from high school to medical school attend the program, and more than 85% have pursued medicine or engineering studies. Professor Lattanza regards this as "probably the most important thing [she] did in [her] career." She is currently the Chair of Orthopaedic Surgery at Yale University, and at UCSF served as Chief of Hand and Upper Extremity Surgery; Fellowship Director; Vice Chair of Diversity, Equity, and Inclusion (DEI); Vice Chair of Faculty Affairs; National Board Member of Shriners; and President of RJOS, among other positions. She also received the AAOS Diversity Award in 2021 for her work with the Perry Initiative among other achievements.

In 2014, Dr Megan Conti Mica, who serves as cochair for the Diversity Committee for the ASSH, was a part of the first female-dominated class of Hand Surgery fellows at Mayo Clinic. She is a part of the first All-Female Hand Surgeons Travel Club, with the aim of mutual mentorship and support.

ON THE SHOULDERS OF WOMEN: NOTABLE NAMES IN HISTORY

In telling the story of female surgeons in upper extremity maladies, the following investigators are highlighted. This list is by no means comprehensive, and the authors regret they could not include all notable names in this article.

Augusta Klumpke: Klumpke Palsy

Dr Dejerine-Klumpke (**Fig. 8**) was a physician and neuroanatomist in the 1800s known for describing lower plexus paralysis and the oculopapillary signs associated with them, a palsy that bears her name.[17,18] Born in San Francisco (1959), she studied medicine in Paris, "where she was a key figure in the development of the French school of neurology that burgeoned in Paris at the turn of the 20th century. She was just 26 years old when she described Klumpke's brachial plexus palsy. Beyond her contributions to neurology, Dr. Déjerine-Klumpke is seen as a pioneer in the history of French feminism, having struggled against prejudice to become the first female intern in Paris. She is also remembered as an innovator in spinal cord injury rehabilitation."[19] For her work as an officer during World War I, she was awarded the French Medal of Recognition and promoted to Officer of the Legion of Honour. She was the first female member (1901), vice president (1913), then president (1914) of the Paris Society of Neurology, and the first female member of the Society of Biology (1923). At 68 years, Dr Klumpke died of breast cancer in Paris, France (1927). "She was a person who did not take no for an answer (Lynda Jun-San Yang, neurosurgeon, University of Michigan), and is the only woman discussed in Boyes'

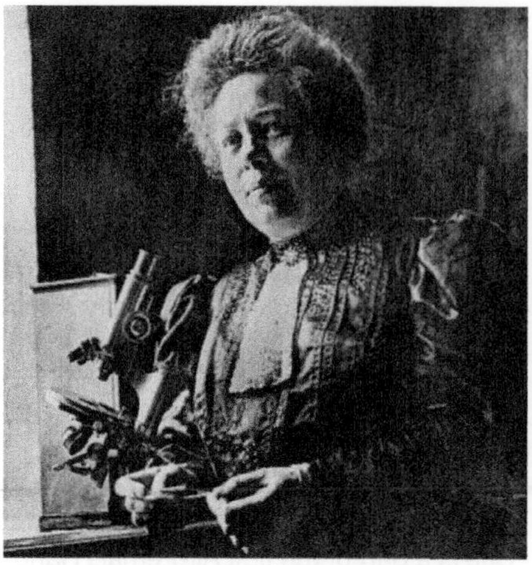

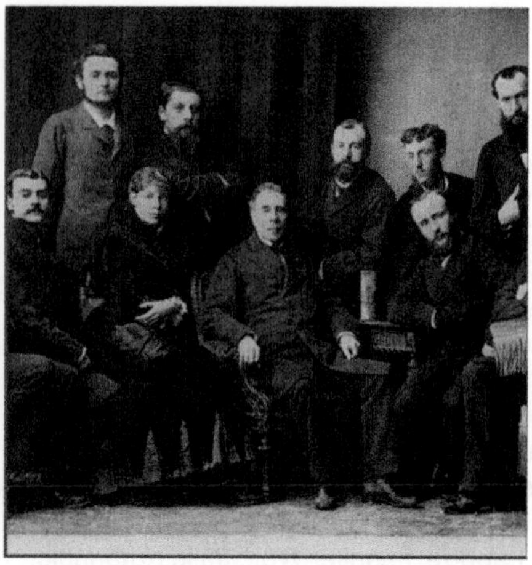

Fig. 8. (*Left*) Dr Augusta Klumpke. (*Right*) 22-Year-old Dr Augusta Klumpke surrounded by male colleagues at a Paris clinic, 1881. (*From* Madame Déjerine 1859-1924 : Déjérine-Klumpke, Augusta Marie, 1859-1927. Internet Archive. Available at https://archive.org/details/b29931630/page/39/mode/2up; and Plate V, La Clinique du Charité, 1881 from "Le Professeur J. Dejerine," 1922. Gauckler, E. Le Professeur J. Dejerine, 1849-1947, by Paris: Masson et Cie, 1922; with permission.)

1976 "On the Shoulders of Giants: Notable Names in Hand Surgery."

Dr Liebe Sokol Diamond: the first woman in the Pediatric Orthaopedic Society of North America

Dr Liebe Sokol Diamond[20–23] (**Fig. 9**) was one of the nation's leading pediatric Orthopedic surgeons and the first female member of Pediatric Orthopaedic Society, and was the 12th board certified female orthopedist in the United States (1964). Born in Baltimore (1931) as a first-generation Jewish immigrant, Dr Sokol Diamond's family was deeply involved in helping Eastern European Jewish refugees resettle in this country.

Dr Sokol Diamond was the first female orthopedic resident at the University of Pennsylvania (1960), hired when she was the only candidate who knew the difference between a cross-cut and a rip saw, distinguishing her from the men. "In retrospect, maybe some of my rough times were because I was a woman," Sokol Diamond said in an interview. "We were tolerated, in a physical sense, but I can't say I was discriminated against in any sense. Out of 200 [interns and residents], there were only five women. You took what was dished out, and you shut up and drank your beer. We all thought that if we made any noise, we'd be kicked out."

Born with multiple hand and foot deformities (amniotic band syndrome), she later started her own congenital practice at the very hospital that had first cared for her. Yet, she never felt this was a limitation—to accommodate her own partial finger amputations, her family commissioned a custom porcelain glove model, from which her surgical gloves were then made.

Her career and research focused on pediatric limb deformities and orthopedic aspects of genetic diseases, where her own anatomy helped patients and parents facing difficult diagnoses and medical situations. "It takes away some of the aloneness...the fear of the future," she said. She was known for her innovative techniques for correcting limb deformities. She also served the State Health Department, the Jewish Family and Children's Society, and was inducted into the Jewish Hall of Fame (2013). Dr Sokol Diamond passed away from leukemia in 2017.

Dr Julia Terzis: Reconstructive Microsurgery and "Babysitter" Procedure

Born in Thessaloniki, Greece, Dr Terzis grew up in post-World War II Salonica. Her father died when she was 5 years old, so her grandmother raised her and her sister while her mother struggled to provide for the family.

Dr Terzis arrived in Pennsylvania in 1961, where she attended university and medical school, before earning her PhD studying neurophysiology of mechanoreceptors from McGill University. She was the first female resident at the Royal Victoria Hospital (Montreal, Canada), one of the birthplaces of microsurgery. She fought to ensure her performance did not reflect poorly on her gender, even returning to work only two days after she gave birth to her only daughter.

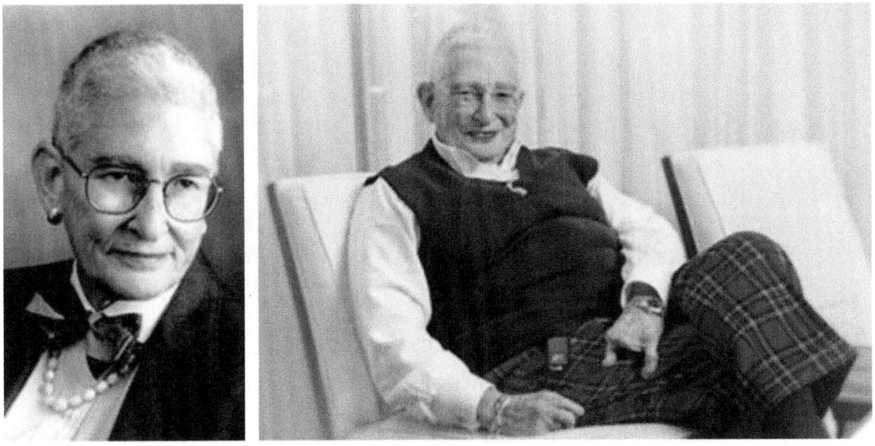

Fig. 9. Dr Liebe Sokol Diamond.

When she rotated through Plastic Surgery, Rollin Daniel and Bruce Williams influenced her to pursue Plastic Surgery and, specifically, Peripheral Nerve surgery. She is recognized worldwide for her vanguard contributions to restorative, reconstructive microsurgery and peripheral nerve paralysis, including involvement in the first neurovascular free flap (1974), the revolutionary concept of the "babysitter" procedure (1984),[24] the first free pectoralis minor muscle for smile restoration, and the first vascularized nerve grafts, and for obstetric brachial plexus injury treatment, the dynamic scapula stabilization procedure, and the selective ipsilateral and contralateral C7 technique.

Dr Terzis (**Figs. 10** and **11**) was a founding member of the International Society for Reconstructive Microsurgery and one of the founders of the American Society for Reconstructive Microsurgery. She has led the Plastic Surgery Research Council (PSRC), the International Microsurgical Society, and the World Society for Reconstructive Microsurgery. Dr Terzis currently resides in New York.[25,26]

Dr. Susan Mackinnon: Translational Research in Nerve Surgery

Born in Campbellton, New Brunswick, Canadian Dr Mackinnon originally planned to be a history teacher.[27,28] After completing medical school, residency, and research in Canada, she trained at the Raymond Curtis Hand Center (Union Memorial Hospital, Baltimore, 1982). In 1984, Dr Mackinnon began experimenting with pretreated nerve allografts and host immunosuppression, and, as she has repeated throughout her career, translated this bench research into clinical applications, reconstructing a child's sciatica nerve in 1988.[24] She also conceived and developed the concept of nerve transfers to reinnervate muscles denervated by injury at a higher level, creating a monumental paradigm shift in how surgeons treat nerve injuries.[14] In addition to publishing hundreds of articles and book chapters, with her colleague Dr Ida Fox, she developed a military-funded Web site to democratize and educate surgeons everywhere in surgical techniques.[29] This content has generated millions of views over hundreds of countries around the world. Dr Mackinnon has also been outspoken in developing female surgeons through role modeling, mentorship, and most importantly, sponsorship. Her life and work have impacted incalculable legions of patients, surgeons, and female physicians, globally.

Dr Mackinnon is the recipient of multiple prestigious awards and leadership positions, including but not limited to, the Gold Medal Award in Surgery by the Royal College of Physicians and Surgeons; fellow of the Institute of Medicine of the National Academy of Sciences; President of AAPS, AAHS, ASPN, and PSRC; AAPS Honorary Award; Clinician of the Year, Research Achievement Award in Basic Science; and Distinguished Fellow. She was awarded the Jacobson award in innovation for the American College of Surgeons. She was the Chief of her division for nearly 25 years before stepping down in 2020. Dr Mackinnon was recently honored as a Pioneer in Hand Surgery by the IFSSH in 2022.

Dr Jacquelin Perry: Mentor and Role Model

Born May 31, 1918, in Colorado Dr Jacquelin Perry (**Fig. 12**) was raised in Los Angeles.[30,31] The daughter of a clothing shop clerk and salesman, she was determined to become a physician from a very young age. She committed herself to reading every textbook in the Los Angeles library from childhood. After receiving her bachelor's degree in Physical Education from the University of

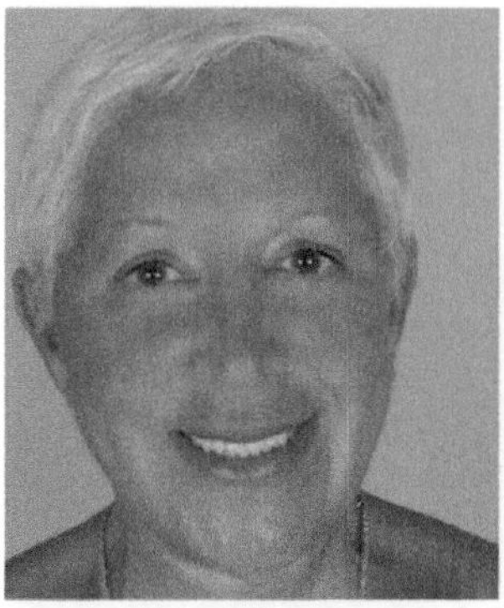

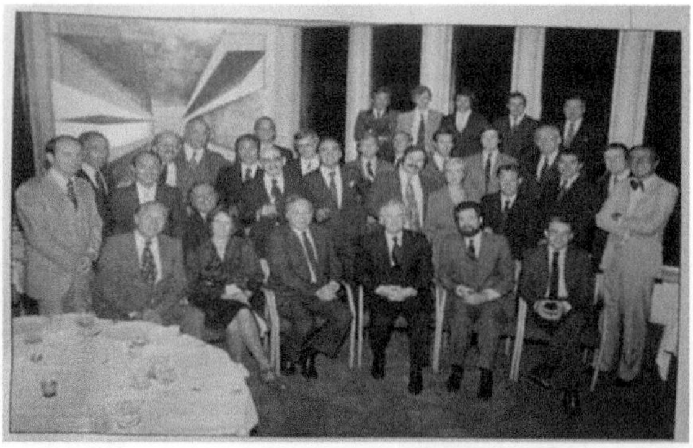

Fig. 10. (*Left*) Dr Julia Terzis. (*Right*) In 1984, the American Society for Reconstructive Microsurgery (ASRM) was established. Photograph of the attendees of the first annual meeting of the ASRM. There are two women: Dr Jane Petro (first row, second from left) and Dr Julia Terzis (second row, seventh from the left).

California Los Angeles (UCLA) in 1940, she joined the US Army and trained as a physical therapist, which gave her a background of working with polio recovery patients. Following World War II, she pursued medicine with the G.I. Bill, and graduated as the first female Orthopedic surgeon from UCSF. Known colloquially as "The Grand Dame of Orthopaedics" she became one of the first ten women certified by the ABOS. The foremost expert in the United States on gait analysis, her research and expertise were founded on decades of working with post-poliomyelitis patients at Los Angeles Rancho Los Amigos Medical Center. The Jacquelin Perry Neuro-Trauma Institute and Rehabilitation Center at Rancho Los Amigos was dedicated in 1996 in her honor, and multiple awards and initiative are named in her honor, including a research award in her name, as well as The Perry Initiative, a national engineering and medicine outreach program responsible for building a pipeline today of women in medicine and engineering. She is responsible for pioneering our current understanding of neuro-orthopedics, functional assist devices, and training leaders in the field of neuro-orthopedics today, including Dr Mary Ann Keenan and Dr Lattanza.

Among the first generation of female Orthopedic surgeons, you would be hard pressed to find one who does not mention Dr Perry as an influence, inspiration, or mentor.

Where Are We Now

A decade ago, the ASSH performed an analysis[15] from 1995 to 2012 regarding ethnic and gender diversity in Hand Surgery trainees. Statistically significant yet minimal linear growth of 0.61%, 0.48%, and 0.66% per year ($P < .05$ for all) was found for proportions of female trainees in Hand, Orthopedic, and Plastic Surgery, respectively. Encouragingly, the proportion of US women in the ASSH has grown from 9.3% in 2010% to 14.3% in 2016, and the percentage of US female presenters at the annual meeting has increased to 15.9%.[32]

A Look to the Future

> *Increased gender diversity correlates with improvement in quality of medical education, research productivity and health care accessibility.*
>
> —*MA Simon, JY Reede*[33,34]

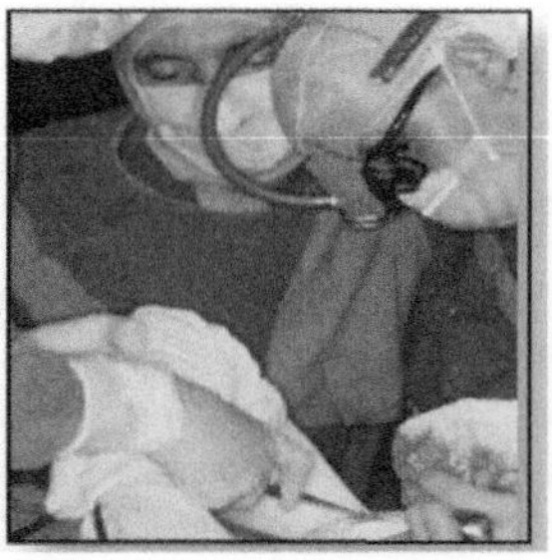

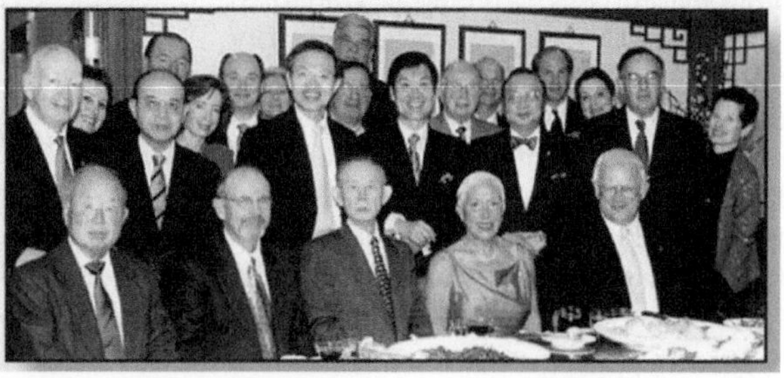

Fig. 11. (*Left*) Dr Terzis (*right*) and Dr Manktelow (*center*) transferring the first pectoralis minor flap at Royal Victoria hospital on January 26, 1981. (*Right*) 2001 Inaugural Congress of the WSRM, Taipei, Taiwan (Dr Terzis is first/lower row, fourth from left).

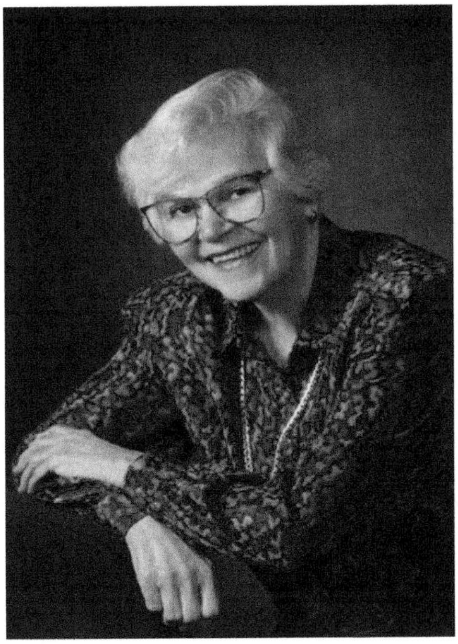

Fig. 12. Dr Jacquelin Perry.

It actually doesn't take much to be considered a difficult woman. That's why there are so many of us.

—Jane Goodall

When I'm sometimes asked when will there be enough [women on the Supreme Court] and I say, 'When there are nine,' people are shocked. But there'd been nine men, and nobody's ever raised a question about that.

—Ruth Bader Ginsburg

Women in medical school, in surgery, and women in Hand Surgery, no matter the pace, are undoubtedly increasing.[35,36] These small incremental gains are not an eventuality; each annual 0.5% (or less) increase represents a Sisyphean and hard-won token of the cumulative grit and emotionally erosive micro/macroaggressions our foremothers have endured. Although times may be changing (slowly), we must not only remember the legacy of female surgeons who have contributed to the profession but also the history of hardship that has not yet earned women complete inclusion and belonging in our specialty. Mindful, intentional sponsorship and abandonment of "othering" behavior can only serve to better our specialty and outcomes for our patients.

We all need friends and mentors - not so much to show the way, but to share the way.

—Marybeth Ezaki

ACKNOWLEDGMENTS

The authors are grateful to the women who generously and courageously shared their time and lived experiences. This is a modest, incomplete representation of what was uncovered through oral history, historical documents, and photographs, about the legacy of female hand surgeons. It is impossible to fully honor the strength, wisdom, and accomplishments of these women. The authors hope this is the first step in future investigations to document the history and impact female surgeons have had on Hand Surgery and on the lives of innumerable patients.

DISCLOSURE

Dr W. Chen is a paid consultant for Allergan for the LIMITLESS initiative for female surgeons. Dr A. Topaz has nothing to disclose.

REFERENCES

1. Wirtzfeld DA. The history of women in surgery. Can J Surg 2009;52(4):317–20. PMID: 19680519; PMCID: PMC2724816.
2. One surgeon's principles. Bulletin of the American College of Surgeons. Available at: https://bulletin.facs.org/2015/05/one-surgeons-principles/. Accessed Jun 15, 2020.
3. Stone Age brain surgery? It might have been more survivable than you think. Dave Davies. Available at: https://www.npr.org/transcripts/1089213668. Accessed May 9, 2022.
4. Steven W, Sutton LP. History of Women in Surgery. 41st Annual Seminar of The American Academy of Cardiovascular Perfusion. Available at: https://www.theaacp.com/wp-content/uploads/2020/04/History-of-Women-In-Surgery.pdf. Grand Sierra Resort, Reno, Nevada. Accessed May 9, 2022.
5. SYM06: Women in Hand Surgery: Challenges We Face. Session Handout. Moderated by Melissa A. : Sonya P. Agnew D, Megan A. Conti M, Erika G. Gantt, MD, and Diane E S. Payne, MD, MPT. 75th Annual Meeting of ASSH, Virtual Meeting. October 1-3, 2020. Available at: https://www.assh.org/annualmeeting/servlet/servlet.FileDownload?file=00P0a00000r9TMyEAM. Accessed May 9, 2022.
6. Mary Edwards Walker. Available at: https://en.wikipedia.org/wiki/Mary_Edwards_Walker. Accessed May 9th,2022.
7. Manring MM, Calhoun JH. Biographical sketch: Ruth Jackson, MD, FACS 1902-1994. Clin Orthop Relat Res 2010;468(7):1736–8. PMID: 20182831; PMCID: PMC2882004.
8. Solomon MP, GHranick MS. Alma Dea Morani, MD: A Pioneer in Plastic Surgery. Ann PRS 1997;38(4):431–6.

9. Carter PR. The embryogenesis of the specialty of Hand Surgery: a story of three great Americans – a politician, a general, and a duck hunter: The 2002 Richard J Smith memorial lecture. J Hand Surg Am 2003;28(2):185–98.
10. Newmeyer William L III, Green David P, George E, et al. American society for surgery of the hand: the first fifty years. New York: Churchill Livingstone; 1995.
11. Alan Freeland Dr. The First Twenty-Five Years, History of the American Association for Hand Surgery. Available at: https://handsurgery.org/multimedia/files/25-Years-History-Book.pdf. Accessed May 9, 2022.
12. The Upper Hand: Chuck & Chris Talk Hand Surgery Interview 3: Marybeth Ezaki. Past ASSH President, Current Mentor and Sage. Published May 10, 2020. Season 1. Episode 18.
13. Bulletin of the University of Maryland School of Medicine 1986-1987. Available at: http://hdl.handle.net/10713/2966. Accessed May 9, 2022.
14. Russel Robert C. History of the American Association for Hand Surgery 1995-2020. Available at: https://handsurgery.org/multimedia/files/History-of-AAHS.pdf. accessed May 9, 2022.
15. Bae GH, Lee AW, Park DJ, Maniwa K, Zurakowski D, ASSH Diversity Committee, Day CS. Ethnic and gender diversity in hand surgery trainees. J Hand Surg Am 2015;40(4):790–7. Epub 2015 Jan 29. PMID: 25639841.
16. Ruth Jackson Orthopedic Society. Available at: http://www.rjos.org. Accessed June 15, 2022.
17. Balakrishnan VS. Augusta Dejerine-Klumpke. Lancet Neurol 2018;17(11):936. Epub 2018 Apr 23. PMID: 29681502.
18. Scientist of the Day: Augusta Klumpke. October 18, 2018. Available at: https://www.lindahall.org/about/news/scientist-of-the-day/augusta-klumpke. Accessed 05-12-2022.
19. Augusta Dijerine-Klumpke, M.D. (1859-1927): A historical perspective on Klumpkes palsy. Neurosurgery 2008;63(2):359–66. ; discussion 366-7. (Sept 2008).
20. Women's History Month Highlight: Dr. Liebe Sokol Diamond. Available at: https://posna.org/News/Women-s-History-Month-Highlight-Dr-Liebe-Sokol-Dia. Accessed May 9, 2022.
21. Legacy of Learning A. Pediatric Residency Program Receives $1 Million Gift from Celebrated Surgeon and Educator Liebe Sokol Diamond, MD. Changing Lives through Philanthropy at LifeBridge Health. Summer 2017 Issue. Available at: https://www.lifebridgehealth.org/Uploads/Public/Documents/Development/ChangingLivesSummer2017.pdf. Accessed June 6, 2022.
22. Pediatric Orthopedic Society of North America. Our Society History. In Memoriam. Liebe Sokol Diamond, MD. 1931-2017. Available at: https://posna.org/Our-Society/History/In-Memoriam?itemid=95. Accessed June 6, 2022.
23. Liebe Diamond MD. An Oral History. Valerie S. Thaler. American Medical Women's Association. Available at: https://www.amwa-doc.org/wp-content/uploads/2017/06/Liebe-Sokol-Diamond-Oral-History.pdf. Accessed June 6, 2022.
24. History of Microsurgery." American Society for Reconstructive Microsurgery. Available at: https://www.microsurg.org/about-asrm/history-of-microsurgery/. Accessed May 9, 2022.
25. The Icon Project. AAPS. Interview on YouTube. Accessed May 9, 2022.
26. Photos from Available at: https://www.wsrm.net/wp-content/uploads/2018/09/2009-Winter-Newsletter.pdf. Accessed May 9, 2022.
27. Mackinnon Susan. Groundbreaking scientist and nerve surgeon. St. Louis Public Radio. By Floria S. Ross. Available at: https://news.stlpublicradio.org/health-science-environment/2011-03-28/susan-mackinnon-groundbreaking-scientist-and-nerve-surgeon. Accessed June 6, 2022.
28. Susan E, Mackinnon MD, FACS FRCSC, et al. Jacobson Innovation Award. American College of surgeons Bulletin. 2013. Available at: https://bulletin.facs.org/2013/08/mackinnon-receives-jacobson-award/. Accessed June 6, 2022.
29. Learn Surgery. Available at: https://surgicaleducation.wustl.edu. Accessed June 6, 2022.
30. Elliott CK, Headley JL. Jacquelin Perry, MD, DSc (Hon). Polioplace, A Service of Post-Polio Health International. Available at: http://www.polioplace.org/people/jacquelin-perry-md-dsc-hon. Accessed June 14th, 2022.
31. Available at: https://www.aoassn.org/pillar-jacquelin-perry/. Accessed June 14, 2022.
32. Earp BE, Mora AN, Rozental TD. Extending a Hand: Increasing Diversity at the American Society for Surgery of the Hand. J Hand Surg Am 2018;43(7):649–56. Epub 2018 May 25. PMID: 29807843.
33. Simon MA. Racial, ethnic, and gender diversity and the resident operative experience. How can the Academic Orthopaedic Society shape the future of orthopaedic surgery? Clin Orthop Relat Res 1999;360:253–9. PMID: 10101332.
34. Reede JY. A recurring theme: the need for minority physicians. Health Aff (Millwood) 2003;22(4):91–3. PMID: 12889755.
35. Grandizio LC, Pavis EJ, Hayes DS, et al. Analysis of Gender Diversity Within Hand Surgery Fellowship Programs. J Hand Surg Am 2021;46(9):772–7. Epub 2021 Jun 7. PMID: 34112545.
36. Brisbin AK, Chen W, Goldschmidt E, et al. Gender Diversity in Hand Surgery Leadership. Hand (N Y). 2022. https://doi.org/10.1177/15589447211038679. 15589447211038679.

Women in Hand Surgery
Considerations and Support

Cathleen Cahill, MD*, Megan Conti Mica, MD

KEYWORDS

• Women in hand surgery • Infertility • Obstetric complications • Work-like balance • Childcare

KEY POINTS

- Female surgeons can face an increased risk of infertility and obstetric complications, and a lack of support during family planning and pregnancy.
- Breastfeeding can be considered a daunting endeavor due to the lack of available resources, time, and negative perceptions of coworkers.
- Surgical residents work approximately 80 h per week, which is often incongruous with daycare hours.

INTRODUCTION

Hand surgery training is rigorous, with its intent to create competent surgeons prepared to appropriately care for their patients. Trainees are faced with an increased risk of infertility and obstetric complications, breastfeeding difficulties, and a lack of perceived support from peers, residency leadership, and nationally from groups like the Accreditation Council for Graduate Medical Education (ACGME). These factors can deter women from pursuing a career in hand surgery or discourage them from family planning during the residency that is traditionally during the peak of women's fertility. Similarly, practicing Hand surgeons face challenges with regard to call, maternity leave policy, and financial burdens. Surgeons should not have to choose between a career and a family.

HISTORY OF WOMEN IN ORTHOPEDICS

Historically, surgical specialties have been considered "male-dominated." The first female physician in the United States was Dr Elizabeth Blackwell, who was rejected from 20 medical schools before being accepted to Geneva Medical College, after which the medical students voted on her acceptance. Her struggle for a career in medicine continued after graduating when she was unable to obtain a residency and worked as a nurse in France. Similarly, the first female surgeon in the United States was Dr Mary Edwards Walker who graduated from medical school in 1855 and was the first female surgeon in the US Army in 1863.[1] Another notable leader in the field of orthopedics was Ruth Jackson, the first female board-certified Orthopedic surgeon in the United States and first female admitted to the American Academy of Orthopedic Surgeons (AAOS). Her legacy in orthopedics lives on in the Ruth Jackson Orthopedic Society, a networking community for female orthopedic trainees and practicing surgeons. The first African American Orthopedic surgeon was Dr Claudia Thomas, who graduated from Yale medical school in 1980. She completed her fellowship at the University of Maryland and was an assistant professor at Johns Hopkins. A titan in the field and advocate for social justice in health care, throughout her career she fought against racial injustice and to increase minority medical students.

BACKGROUND

To become a board-certified Hand surgeon, one must complete medical school, a residency program in either Orthopedic Surgery, plastic and reconstructive surgery, or general surgery with

UChicago Medicine and Biological Sciences, 5841 South Maryland Avenue, MC3079, Chicago, IL 60637, USA
* Corresponding author.
E-mail address: Cathleen.cahill@uchospitals.edu

Hand Clin 39 (2023) 65–72
https://doi.org/10.1016/j.hcl.2022.08.013
0749-0712/23/Published by Elsevier Inc.

plastic and reconstructive surgery fellowship. At minimum, this is a decade long dedication during the peak of childbearing years. The average American female gives birth to their first child at the age of 26, whereas trainees graduate from their residency programs around the age of 32.[2]

Diversity Statistics

Fifty years ago, in plastic and reconstructive surgery programs, about 2% of Plastic Surgery residents were female. Similarly, orthopedic surgery has suffered from a lack of female representation. At present, orthopedic surgery continues to have the lowest female recruitment of all surgical subspecialties.[3] Now, about half of medical students are female and diversity in Orthopedic Surgery and Plastic Surgery training programs is a goal. Approximately 38.1% of Plastic Surgery residents are female.[4] Currently, 6% of Orthopedic surgeons and 16% of orthopedic surgery trainees are female.[5] In a large survey of women in orthopedic residency and practice, the most common reasons cited for having chosen orthopedics were enjoyment of manual tasks, professional satisfaction, and intellectual stimulation.[6] Most programs lack the initiative to support female residents creating this sluggish growth in diversity.

The gender disparity in Orthopedic and Plastic Surgery training programs is likely multifactorial, some studies cite implicit gender bias and the negative stigma associated with a pregnant female as a possible reason for lack of female representation.[7] Some major assumptions about orthopedic surgery include the uncontrollable and busy lifestyle intrinsic to the specialty that prohibits a sustainable work–life balance, the necessity of immense physical strength, the “jock fraternity” or “old boys club” culture, and gender-based discrimination.[8] For medical students choosing a career, these assumptions not only discourage women from entering the field of orthopedics, but also negatively impact current female orthopedic trainees when it comes to family planning, maternity, and childcare. In one survey study, female trainees were more likely to delay starting a family until after training, which could arise later issues with infertility.[4]

Female Faculty

In leadership positions, women represent 9% of tenured professors, 12% of department chairs, and 11% of US medical school deans.[9] Based on the current growth rate of 2% per year it will take approximately 217 years for orthopedic surgery to achieve gender parity with the overall medical profession.[10] This emphasizes the need for additional support for women in orthopedics. There is more to be done with respect to acknowledging barriers and accommodating for female surgeons. Encouraging females into the male-dominated surgical specialties is one step, but similarly the workplace itself must change to accommodate this changing demographic. Some proposed solutions include mentorship and sponsorship programs for females, clear maternity leave policies, flexible work hours, lactation room convenience, and on-site childcare. The culture of surgical training and surgical practices is changing, and with it—the experience of the surgeon's mother.

At the faculty level, male and female Orthopedic surgeons in faculty leadership positions have similar research productivity. Despite this similarity in academic productivity, there still exists a large discrepancy in leadership positions.[11] In one study of 160 residency programs, women comprised 13.9% of assistant professors, 10.8% of associate professors, and 1.4% of department chair.[11] Furthermore, women in academic medicine are promoted at slower rates than men and are less likely to hold tenured academic positions. In one study, women in academic medicine felt they were not recognized or rewarded appropriately for their measurable accomplishments when compared with men in the same positions.[12] A possible theory for this disparity would be a perceived burden of balancing familial and household responsibilities during a time of career development. Other proposed ideas are that women are less likely to have mentors and sponsors who push for their career advancement. Lack of mentorship is a possible cause of the lack of female representation in Orthopedic Surgery. Programs with greater numbers of female faculty had larger numbers of female trainees, suggesting mentorship as a way to increase the recruitment of female trainees.[13]

INFERTILITY

In the past, the experience of a pregnant female hand surgery trainee has been challenging. Deferring childbearing until after residency can be an enticing option-with increased salary and more predictable, flexible hours. Waiting until training completion can avoid graduation delay, prevent guilt associated with burdening coworkers with extra work, and inhibit negative perceptions of the pregnant resident. However, wage loss during maternity leave while still being expected to support monthly overhead can be costly once in practice, on top of the medical bills associated with childbirth, possible lack of support from colleagues or not making a partner can create different yet equally stressful risks to having children once in practice. Ultimately, there is no perfect time to have children during one's career.

However, for most trainees, residency takes place during prime reproductive years. The average female hand surgery trainee completes residency at age 31 and enters hand fellowship training. Therefore, females need to be educated about the impact surgical training may have on fertility, childbearing, breastfeeding, and family planning. For many residents and practicing surgeons, the decision to defer childbearing until after training can be difficult due to the age-related fertility decline. Trainees may consider fertility preservation or desire infertility treatment. Infertility is defined as the inability to conceive after 1 year of regular unprotected sexual intercourse for women younger than 35 years of age and after 6 months for women older than 35 years of age. In one study of 327 US female physicians, 24% of respondents reported infertility.[14] The probability of pregnancy is twice as high for women aged 19 to 26 years compared with women aged 35-39 years.[15] Average age at first pregnancy in a survey of female Plastic and Reconstructive surgeons was 30.3 years of age $\pm$ 3.6 years. At age 35 a woman is considered to be of advanced maternal age (AMA). A pregnant woman with AMA is considered a geriatric pregnancy, with an inherent increased risk for miscarriage, low birth weight, gestational diabetes, chromosomal and abnormalities, congenital anomalies, and neonatal mortality.[16,17] Delaying pregnancy until completion of training may not be a realistic expectation for many surgeons.

Furthermore, there is a pervasive lack of strong support for our female surgeons by leadership both on a residency level and by the academies of Orthopedic surgery and Plastic surgery. The discussion, transparency, and formal policy is lacking. In a 2019 survey of 299 program directors (PDs), over half of PDs (55.2%) estimated less than 5% of their residents were facing recurrent pregnancy loss or infertility.[15] This prediction is staggeringly low based on recent survey responses of female physicians. The most common resources offered to surgical trainees were moral support from PDs, time off for appointments, and insurance coverage.[15] However, this is the tip of the iceberg of support that is needed by our female surgeons. This includes infertility support, family planning resources, access to lactation rooms, time off for child care and postpartum along with support for affordable childcare.

FERTILITY PRESERVATION

For surgical trainees who wish to defer childbearing, oocyte cryopreservation has been used by increasing numbers of surgical trainees. In one survey, only 5% of Plastic Surgery trainees underwent oocyte cryopreservation. In a survey PDs, 55% of PDs felt their program's support level was aligned with their personal support for residents undergoing fertility preservation. However, 19% of PDs felt the program was less supportive.[15]

This procedure can offer the busy female resident an option for childbearing in a delayed fashion. However, this procedure can be timely, unsuccessful, expensive, and often painful. It involves hormonal injections, frequent labs, and multiple ultrasounds to ensure optimal egg maturation. These procedures are not conducive to a busy surgeon practice with an unpredictable schedule. A woman undergoing the harvesting process needs flexibility provided by leadership to allow a focus on her medical needs. In addition, the process of egg retrieval involves risks to neurovascular structures and other complications. It is a daunting and costly process to consider that is generally not covered by insurance and is estimated to cost \$10,000–\$20,000 with storage fees of \$300–\$500 per year.[18,19]

For women pursuing in vitro fertilization, the percentage of in vitro fertilization cycles that result in a baby declines from about 40% for women aged 32 and younger, to about 20% for 40-year-old women.[11] Infertility is an acutely painful reality for many surgeons and surgical trainees. A supportive environment for female residents pursuing fertility preservation is crucial. Flexible hours and time for doctors' appointments may ease the toll of fertility preservation amidst training and practice.

OBSTETRICAL COMPLICATIONS

Female Orthopedic surgeons are twice as likely to suffer from complications during pregnancy as women in the general population (31% vs 15% respectively).[20] In one survey, female plastic surgery trainees reported a complication rate of four times the general population. Complications during pregnancy were reported in 56.6% of female plastic surgery trainees.[21] The most common complication was hyperemesis gravidarum, which was experienced by 16.7% of female plastic surgery trainees, the second most common being preterm labor.[22] Obstetric complications place significant stress on the female surgeon, compounded by the stress associated with time away from practice or for surgeons in training away from crucial educational experiences and in some cases, delay in completion of training. The practicing Hand surgeon faces challenges related to call burden, guilt of redirecting patient care, and ease of transition to full-time practicing surgeon.

Knowledge of these obstetric complications can be discouraging for surgeons who wish to become pregnant. Specifically, long hours within the work week, sleep deprivation, >6 h a day spent on ones' feet may can place undue stress.

Effect of Stress

Physical and emotional stress is often encountered in the pregnant surgeon. Often, they must rely on their colleagues for support. For some pregnant residents, the stress associated with burdening coworkers can be as daunting as the stress associated with carrying a heavy workload. Therefore, residents are hesitant to share the load to avoid the guilt of burdening a coworker. A pregnant woman's stress has been shown to cause catecholamine release that could negatively impact the pregnancy. In a study by Holzman and colleagues,[23] in midpregnancy higher levels of urinary catecholamines were associated with a greater risk of spontaneous preterm delivery. In addition, women who underwent premature delivery were found to have elevated levels of inflammatory cytokines in amniotic fluid.[24]

Work hours

In one survey of 1020 female surgeons, there was an increased risk of preterm labor and preterm delivery among women who reported working more than 60 h per week.[20] Therefore, reducing the work hours and night call for pregnant residents is an important consideration. In addition, long work hours upright in the operating room can cause postural alterations in uterine blood flow which can lead to increased uterine contractility and potentially, preterm labor.[25]

Effects of Sleep on Pregnancy

For most surgeons, sleep is a last priority when it comes to balancing a heavy workload and familial responsibilities. Sleep deprivation has been shown to increase the risk of errors and workplace accidents, as well as cause metabolic abnormalities that can negatively affect a developing fetus.[26] The National Sleep Foundation recommends 7-8 h of sleep in a 24-h period for the average adult. Chronic sleep deprivation impairs glucose and fat metabolism and increases inflammatory processes. As a result, cognitive functioning is impaired, and job performance, mental health, and overall quality of life suffers.[26]

Unfortunately, there is an increased risk of prolonged labor and higher rate of cesarean births when averaging less than 6 h of sleep per night during the last month of pregnancy.[27] For medicine trainees, one-half of female residents averaged at least one night per week without sleep during the first and second trimesters, and 44% averaged one night per week without sleep during the third trimester.[28] In addition, women residents experience a higher rate of preterm labor and preeclampsia compared with the wives of their male co-residents.[29] In one study of 19 healthy women, higher levels of pro-inflammatory cytokines were found in women who reported short sleep duration and poor sleep efficiency in mid- and late-pregnancy. Furthermore, the rate of obstetrical complications among residents who had up to six nights on call per month (26.4%) was significantly lower than those who had more than six nights on call per month (49.3%).[22] These are similar effects one would expect with attending surgeons who participate in surgeries and workweeks without any work hour restrictions.

Effect of Operating Hours

For trainees and practicing Hand surgeons, the workday often consists of several surgeries in which the surgeon may or may not be able to sit. Long hours standing in the operating room, whereas often wearing heavy lead for radiation protection, is considered as a physiologic stressor in pregnant residents. In one study, operating more than 8 h per week was associated with an increased risk of obstetric complications in pregnant residents.[22] Unfortunately due to the strenuous demands of being an Orthopedic surgeon, 23.2% of pregnancies are associated with activity restriction, and 10% associated with bedrest.[30]

Occupational Hazards

Some Orthopedic surgeons are exposed to ionizing radiation on a regular basis (several times a week to daily), with fluoroscopy being a frequently used tool for intraoperative fracture care. Ionizing radiation has the greatest detrimental effects on a developing fetus at 3-8 weeks. Though there are no clear limitations on radiation exposure, the American Obstetricians and Gynecologists Committee Opinion states that <5 rads is not harmful to the fetus. However, cumulative doses of radiation are associated with higher rates of childhood cancer. To decrease radiation exposure, surgeons wear lead aprons. However, these are costly, ranging from several hundred to thousands of dollars. For many residency programs, cost coverage is not provided for personal lead aprons. Therefore, female residents are forced to either cover the cost themselves or use hospital-owned, scarce, and often ill-fitting lead aprons. Also, maternity lead aprons are heavier than standard and can be rather uncomfortable to wear during long surgeries.

For trainees and practicing surgeons, occupational hazards place the pregnant surgeon at undue risk. Percutaneous injury can lead to bloodborne exposure to Hepatitis C, Hepatitis A, and human immunodeficiency virus. These viruses have possibility of vertical exposure and postexposure prophylaxis may be detrimental to a breastfeeding infant or fetus.[30] In addition, nitrous oxide and other anesthetic gases can cause chromosomal abnormalities. Methylmethacrylate (MMA), commonly used in bone cement, is a known to be associated with fetotoxicity and the Environmental Protection Agency recommends exposure level <1000 ppm over an 8-h period based on animal studies.[30] Accommodations need to be made to minimize exposure to these dangers. Absence during intubation and extubation of patients and cementing of prosthesis is an option for pregnant surgeons though may not be realistic.

BREASTFEEDING

Returning to work after childbirth can be a very difficult period. Physicians are burdened with new family responsibilities on top of clinical duties. Breastfeeding during can be considered a daunting endeavor due to lack of available resources, time, and negative perceptions of coworkers.

Breastfeeding postpartum is mutually beneficial for both mother and baby. Mothers experience less postpartum blood loss, and lower rates of postpartum depression, diabetes, and breast and ovarian cancer. Infant benefits include decreased rates of allergies, infections, obesity, and sudden infant death syndrome. It has also been shown to improve neurodevelopment and provide gastrointestinal benefits for infants.[31]

Despite these proven benefits, lactating surgeons are more likely to stop breastfeeding or pumping earlier than intended. In one survey of Plastic Surgery residents, female trainees were dissatisfied with the length of time breastfeeding.[4] The average duration of breastfeeding was training 4.7 months vs. 8.3 months. Inability to breastfeed one's child for the desired duration is often due to workplace time constraints and lack of privacy. Professional pressure to maintain the same workload before maternity leave results in inflexible schedules and inability to take the necessary time to expel milk from breasts. On average breastfeeding or pumping adds as average of 35 h per week without built-in pump breaks during the clinic and operating days, surgeons may experience mastitis and loss of milk supply. In addition, access to proper location rooms with a locked door and appropriate arrangements continues to be a problem despite laws set in place nationwide. Location can be hard and add the lack of support or accommodations for these working mothers, their personal goals cannot be met by the demands of their professional goals. There is no reason these goals need to be mutually exclusive.

In a survey of PDs from 2000, 20% defined allowances for breastfeeding on return to clinical duties. Furthermore, of 178 ACGME accredited orthopedic surgery programs, only 2.8% had written breastfeeding policies available for review on the orthopedic surgery residency-specific website.[31] In this same study, dedicated lactation facilities were listed as available for only 1.7% of programs. Accessible and available lactation rooms in the workplace and clear information regarding breastfeeding policies would certainly ease the transition from maternity leave to full-time surgeon and parent. In addition, making a clear and visible policy would assist in normalizing breastfeeding or pumping during the workday. Without stated and visible policy and convenient lactation rooms, physicians and coworkers may view breastfeeding as abnormal behavior or a workplace inconvenience. In one study, 82% of surgical trainees reported being uncomfortable asking attending surgeons for permission to step away from the operating room to regularly express milk.[7] Trainees and surgeons alike need to feel empowered to take time to breastfeed, and formal policy with accessible lactation facilities, not bathrooms, would be beneficial.

MATERNITY LEAVE POLICY

Experience of Maternity Leave in Training

The American Council of Graduate Medical Education (ACGME) starting July 1, 2022 required all ACGME accredited programs to offer 6 weeks of paid leave for all residents and fellows for medical, parental, and caregiver leave. Before this update, the ACGME did not have specific leave requirements, only that "the contract/agreement must contain or provide a reference for leave."[32] To put this in perspective, women who deliver via Cesarean section are told to refrain from lifting anything heavier than her baby for 6 weeks. With most women taking 4 to 6 weeks of maternity leave, they are pressured to disregard their own postoperative restrictions to rejoin the workforce—putting themselves at increased risk.[33]

Previously, there was significant variability in the duration of maternity leave in orthopedic surgery training, and the AAOS did not provide a standardized policy for parental leave. Based on a survey of plastic and reconstructive surgery residents, the mean maternity leave during training was 5.5 weeks. 62.2% of residents were unhappy with the amount of maternity of leave they took and 47% of trainees reported that their program had a formal maternity leave policy.[4]

In a 2017 survey of 88 Plastic and Reconstructive surgery PDs in the United States, 38% of respondents reported their program had a maternity leave policy. Of the programs that did not have maternity leave policies, 26% believed a maternity leave policy would leave to gaps in resident training, and 12% reported a small class size would lead to insufficient workload coverage.[34]

In a survey of 2188 general surgery and surgical subspecialty residents examining the perception of parental leave in the United States, about one-third of residents, regardless of sex, reported that they did not feel supported when they took parental leave.[35]

There have been recent updates allowing more flexible requirements to complete surgical training. The American Board of Orthopedic Surgeons (ABOS) time requirement to sit for boards is 46 weeks per year averaged over 5 years with a minimum completion of 1000 cases over the course of training.[36] The American Board of Plastic Surgery (ABPS) requires a minimum of 5 years of general surgery training followed by three years of Plastic Surgery training, or 6 years of training at an integrated Plastic Surgery program with maternity leave taken when necessary and not just during elective time.[37]

Maternity Leave in Practice

In addition to the previously stated dangers of a truncated maternity leave, there exists a significant financial burden for women Hand surgeons in practice. The average cost for the practicing surgeon is $45,350. It is estimated that each additional week of unpaid leave costs the surgeon $3,252.[38] Also, in certain practices, women surgeons remain responsible for the cost of overhead expenses. With building a new practice, women surgeons are significantly impacted by loss of financial stability and times of decreased practice growth. The average surgeon in practice takes 9.6 weeks of maternity leave. If they take leave before their first year in practice, they may not have short-term disability to support them and protect their job. In addition, this may impact their ability to make partner and revenue to support their building overhead and medical bills alike. The call during maternity leave is generally considered burdensome by partners that add stress on the pregnant surgeon to work double the call before delivery or postpartum. Either scenario adds extra undue stress on the pregnant or postpartum mother that can easily be avoided with a more tolerant and accepting culture adapted by orthopedic surgeons and a collaboration to support female surgeons.

CHILDCARE

Surgeons work about unpredictable and long hours, which is often incongruous with daycare hours. It is difficult to obtain convenient, affordable, and reliable childcare that is forgiving of a surgeon's long and changing hours. Although on call or during a regular workday, unforeseen changes in childcare can cause residents and attendings schedule adjustments or cancelations. Access to affordable and flexible childcare can be a obstacle to career progression and could be one possible reason for less women in leadership positions or end up leaving medicine early in their careers. For few lucky trainees, a village of family, partners or friends can share childcare responsibilities.

There has been a call for on-site childcare which some institutions provide; however, this is the minority. This allows convenient drop-off and pick-up, along with hours that better align with the parents whose children attend the childcare center. This direct access and support by the institution provides stability for surgeons while showing buy-in for their working mothers.

Other options include preferential daycare enrollment, monetary support for childcare or work hour, or access to backup daycare services. Allowing clinic hours and operating room block time around daycare hours helps alleviate some of the stress but understanding this fine balance and importance of the surgeon's personal life is monumental for building a long-term commitment.

WORK–LIFE BALANCE

Now, more than ever, work–life balance has become a reason to choose one career over another. In a 2016 survey of corporate life by Deloitte, 16.8% of millennials surveyed evaluated career opportunities by good work–life balance, 13.4% work for opportunities to progress, and 11% seek flexibility (remote working and flexible hours). Family and professional success are not mutually exclusive. There is a perception that a career in Orthopedic Surgery would be more difficult for a woman to balance than a man. This may be due to the increased household responsibilities women hold over men at home, in general women spend nine more hours a week on household duties. This can be overwhelming. Mentorship and sponsorship are very important in creating a successful balance of work and life. Navigating how to say no to experiences that may not be valuable long term and helping push career propelling opportunities that are focused and will allow career and personal life to co-exist. Work–life balance is possible, it takes to support and a culture change that allows women to still be successful while prioritizing all the aspects of their life that provides meaning and fulfillment.

DISCUSSION

As female representation increases in orthopedics so should the support for the pregnant trainee and practicing surgeon. There is a lack of policy with respect to breastfeeding and childcare. There are cultural barriers such as a lack of perceived support from faculty or leadership. There is the guilt of burdening co-residents during periods of time away. There is an increased risk of infertility and obstetric complications. Therefore, changes in culture and policy to facilitate pregnancy and parenthood in the training program and workplace will help to recruit the best hand surgery trainees, maintain the surgical workforce, promote the well-being of trainees and practicing surgeons, and facilitate success.

REFERENCES

1. Wirtzfeld DA. The history of women in surgery. Can J Surg 2009;52(4):317–20.
2. Goldberg E. When the surgeon is a mom. Available at: www.nytimes.com/2019/12/20/science/doctors-surgery-motherhood-medical-school.html. Accessed April 30, 2020.
3. Chambers CC, Ihnow SB, Monroe EJ, et al. Women in orthopedic surgery, population trends in trainees and practicing surgeons. J Bone Joint Surg Am 2018;100(17):e116.
4. Bourne DA, Chen W, Schilling BK, et al. The impact of plastic surgery training on family planning and prenatal health. Plast Reconstr Surg 2019. https://doi.org/10.1097/PRS.0000000000006100.
5. Scarpella TA, Spiker AM, Lee CA, et al. Next steps: advocating for women in orthopedic surgery. J Am Acad Orthop Surg 2022;30(8):377–86.
6. Rhode RS, Wolf JM, Adams JE. Where are the women in orthopaedic surgery? Clin Orthop Relat Res 2016;474(9):1950–6.
7. Rangel EL, Lyu H, Haider AH, et al. Factors associated with residency and career dissatisfaction in childbearing surgical residents. JAMA Surg 2018; 153(11):1004–11.
8. LaPorte DM, Tornetta P, Marsh JL. Challenges to orthopedic surgery resident education. J Am Acad Orthop Surg 2019;27(12):419–25.
9. Thompson Burdine JA, Telem DA, Waljee JF, et al. Defining barriers and facilitators to advancement for women in academic surgery. JAMA Netw Open 2019;2(8):e1910228.
10. Acuna AJ, Sato EH, Jella TK, et al. How long will it take to reach gender parity in orthopedic surgery in the United States? An analysis of the national provider identifier registry. Clin Orthop Relat Res 2021; 479(6):1179–89.
11. Hoof M.A., Sommi C., Meyer L.E., et al., Gender-related Differnces in Research Productivity, Position, and Advanced Among Academic Orthopedic Faculty Within the United States, J Am Acad Orthop Surg, 28 (21), 2020, 893-899.
12. Murphy M, Callander JK, Dohan D. Women's experience of promotion and tenure in academic medicine and potential implications for gender disparities in career avancement, a qualitative analysis. JAMA Netw Open 2021;4(9):e2125843.
13. Sobel AD, Cox RM, Ashinsky B, et al. Analysis of factors related to the sex diversity of orthopaedic residency programs in the United States. J Bone Joint Surg Am 2018;100(11):e79.
14. Stentz NC, Griffith KA, Perkins E, et al. Fertility and childbearing among american female physicians. J Women's Heal 2016. https://doi.org/10.1089/jwh.2015.5638.
15. Dunson DB, Colombo B, Baird DD. Changes with age in the level and duration of fertility in the menstrual cycle. Hum Reprod 2002;17(5):1399–403.
16. Correa-de-Araujo R, Yoon SS. Clinical outcomes in high rish pregnancies due to advanced maternal age. J Womens Health (Larchmt) 2021;30(2): 160–7.
17. Huynh M, Wang A, Ho J, et al. Fertility preservation and infertility treatment in medical training: an assessment of residency and fellowship program directors' attitudes. Women's Heal Rep 2021;2(1): 576–85.
18. Shupac J., Motherhood postponed: freeze now, hatch later. Canadian Business 2013, Available: www.canadianbusiness.com/economy/motherhood-postponed/. Accessed December 12, 2014.
19. Petropanagos A. Social egg freezing: risk, benefits and other considerations. CMAJ 2015;187(9):666–9.
20. Hamilton AR, Tyson MD, Braga JA, et al. Childbearingand pregnancy characteristics of female orthopaedic sur-geons. J Bone Joint Surg Am 2012;94:e77.
21. Eskenazi L, Weston J. The pregnant plastic surgical resident: results of a survey of women plastic surgeons and plastic surgery residency directors. Plast Reconstr Surg 1995;95(2):330–5.
22. Behbehani S, Tulandi T. Obstetrical complications in pregnant medical and surgical residents. J Obstet

Gynaecol Can 2015. https://doi.org/10.1016/S1701-2163(15)30359-5.

23. Holzman C, Senagore P, Tian Y, et al. Maternal catecholamine levels in midpregnancy and risk of preterm delivery. Am J Epidemiol 2009;170(8):1014–24.
24. Arntzen KJ, Kjollesdal AM, Halgunset J, et al. TNF, IL-1, IL-6, IL-8 and soluble TNF receptors in rela
25. Katz VL, Miller NH, Bowes WA Jr. Pregnancy complicationsof physicians. West J Med 1988;149:704–7.
26. Chang JJ, Pien GW, Duntley SP, et al. Sleep deprivation during pregnancy and maternal and fetal outcomes: Is there a relationship? Sleep Med Rev 2010;14(2):107–14.
27. Lee KA, Zaffke ME, McEnany G. Parity and sleep patterns during and after pregnancy. Obstet Gynecol 2000. https://doi.org/10.1016/S0029-7844(99)00486-X.
28. Osborn LM, Harris DL, Reading JC, et al. Outcome of pregnancies experienced during residency. J Fam Pract 1990;31(6):618–22.
29. Klebanoff MA, Shiono PH, Rhoads GG. Outcomes of pregnancy in a national sample of resident physicians. N Engl J Med 1990;323(15):1040–5.
30. Wessel L., Mulcahey M., Sutton K., The pregnant ortopedic surgeon; risks and precautions, AAOS Now, 2018. Available at: https://www.aaos.org/aaosnow/2018/feb/managing/managing01/.
31. Wynn M, Caldwell L, Kowalski H, et al. Identifying barriers: current breastfeeding policy in orthopedic surgery residency. Iowa Orthop J 2021;41(1):5–9.
32. Accreditation Council For Graduate Medical Education: ACGME common program requirements (residency). Available at: www.acgme.org/Portals/0/PFAssets/ProgramRequirements/CPRResidency2019.pdf. Accessed April 30, 2020.
33. Dwyer E. and Conti Mica M., Antiquated maternity leave policies can deter med students, AAOS Now, Oct 2020. Available at: www.aaosnow.org.
34. Garza RM, Weston JS, Furnas HJ. Pregnancy and the plastic surgery resident. Plast Reconstr Surg 2017. https://doi.org/10.1097/PRS.0000000000002861.
35. Altieri MS, Salles A, Bevilacqua LA, et al. Perceptions of surgery residents about parental leave during training. JAMA Surg 2019. https://doi.org/10.1001/jamasurg.2019.2985.
36. Wright RW, Armstrong AD, Azar FM, et al. The american board of orthopaedic surgery response to COVID-19. J Am Acad Orthop Surg 2020;28(11):e465–8.
37. American Board of Plastic Surgery: Personal Leave Policy. Available at: www.abplasticsurgery.org/media/18074/personal-leave-policy-final-3-19-20.pdf. Accessed June 3, 2020.
38. Nguyen CV, Luong M, Weiss JM, et al. The cost of maternity leave for the orthopaedic surgeon. J Am Acad Orthop Surg 2020;28(22):e1001–5.

The Underrepresented Minority in Hand Surgery

Challenges and Strategy for Success

Marvin Dingle, MD[a], Michael G. Galvez, MD[b,*]

KEYWORDS

- Underrepresented minority • Hand surgery • Diversity

KEY POINTS

- The number of underrepresented minority (underrepresented in medicine [UIM]) Hand surgeons remains incredibly low compared with the diverse population of the United States.
- Each step of the training process to become a Hand surgeon is a potential barrier that a UIM Hand surgeon must face.
- A strategy that identifies the many challenges and considerations for entering Hand Surgery are provided.
- Successful advancement as a medical student, resident, fellow, and attending with mentorship/sponsorship will increase the number of UIM Hand surgeons for the United States.

INTRODUCTION

Hand surgery is a rewarding subspecialty that helps patients get back to living their daily lives, from a child being able to play outside to an adult being able to get back to work. This article serves to identify the challenges that an underrepresented in medicine (UIM) student will face and provide a strategy for identifying resources and important milestones for pursuing a career in Hand Surgery in the United States.

In addition to the academic rigor and personal sacrifices that many students experience, a UIM student's journey is made more difficult by being a gender and/or racial minority. It is not a hyperbole to say that these barriers and challenges begin at an early age. Disparities that affect minority populations can be traced to the zip code of birth or childhood. Racial minorities in the United States face systemic and institutional challenges from health care access to unequal treatment by law enforcement and the judicial system. The authors are no exception to this reality having experienced their own racial prejudices throughout their childhoods and medical training.

Reading the current state of disparities in surgical training can be very discouraging. Accounts of microaggressions, being the "only," always needing to be a "pioneer," and high attrition rates are exhausting to learn and hear about. The lack of UIM mentors and surgeons in leadership positions contribute to the sense that one does not belong in Hand Surgery. Research on racial and gender demographics over the past decades have not shown much improvement in racial diversity of surgical residents and practicing surgeons. Although Hand Surgery has seen a modest increase in gender diversity—14.3% women in 2016, racial diversity has not improved much for African American, Hispanic/Latino, and Native American membership in the American Association for Hand Surgery (ASSH) at 1.7%, 4.3%, and 0% respectively, in 2016.[1]

[a] Department of Surgery, Uniformed Services University of Health Sciences, Walter Reed National Military Medical Center, 8901 Wisconsin Avenue, Bethesda, MD 20889, USA; [b] Division of Plastic and Hand Surgery, Pediatric Hand and Upper Extremity Surgery, Valley Children's Healthcare, 9300 Valley Children's Place GE07, Madera, CA 93636, USA
* Corresponding author.
E-mail address: michaelgalvez@gmail.com

Hand Clin 39 (2023) 73–78
https://doi.org/10.1016/j.hcl.2022.08.004

The authors believe that Hand Surgery provides a tremendously fulfilling career with amazing financial, personal, and social/societal benefits. They believe that the lack of diversity should not hinder a student's desire to want to become a Hand surgeon and contribute to his/her local community—defining success for the UIM individual reading this article. Research demonstrates that with patient's and physician's racial and gender concordance, patients are more likely to adhere to physician instructions and therefore more successful outcomes.[2–4] Perseverance to enter this field is worthwhile.

Why Hand Surgery: The Secret Is Out

Hand surgery is unique and includes incredible breadth, and therefore additional training is warranted (**Fig. 1**). The field encompasses a variety of practice settings which can include academic, group practice, and private practice. Depending on the practice setting, the field includes hand trauma from replantation to mangled extremity, microsurgery, arthritis surgery, reconstructive surgery, congenital hand differences, peripheral nerve injury, brachial plexus injuries, and so forth. To become a Hand surgeon, one must complete either an orthopedic, Plastic Surgery or general surgery residency and then engage an additional 1-year fellowship in Hand Surgery. Aside from becoming board certified in their primary board, Hand surgeons also obtain a certification of the subspecialty of surgery of the hand. Each of these residencies varies in training length from 5 to 7 years. These specialties are competitive compared with some nonsurgical specialties. Plastic surgery and orthopedic surgery are among the most competitive specialties to match into.[5] Please note that general surgery is a pathway to become a Hand surgeon after fellowship; however, this is infrequent compared with orthopedic and Plastic Surgery. There are many orthopedic and Plastic surgeons who practice some aspects of Hand Surgery after completing their residency; however, additional training including the board certification process promotes further subspecialization to occur and therefore more comfort to practice in this complex field.

Similar to investigating any field of medicine or surgery, it becomes important to fully explore Hand Surgery. This includes seeking out shadowing opportunities both in the clinic and the operating room. The goal is to discover what the basic "bread and butter" cases are and what the complex cases are. Experiencing both simple and complex hand and upper extremity surgeries will allow you to appreciate the anatomy and the form and function. If these experiences speak to you, then it becomes important to explore exactly how to pursue this field as a career.

Medical School: Choose Your Adventure

Medical school is a wonderful opportunity to differentiate yourself in Hand Surgery. By shadowing and choosing your field of choice, which typically includes orthopedics and Plastic Surgery, at that point you focus on pursuing your specific residency. The details on how to pursue specific residencies are beyond the scope of this article. Here, we hope to demonstrate that finding the love for Hand Surgery can happen early. The earlier you differentiate into a Hand surgeon, the sooner you can shoot for the goal of matching into a hand fellowship to become a Hand surgeon.

Although gender demographics of medical school matriculants in the United States have improved greatly over the past few years, the representation of students from racial minority backgrounds has changed minimally.[6] There have been large strides in gender representation in medical school with nearly half of all medical schools being women. However, African American and Hispanic/Latino and Alaskan/Native students have seen minimal improvements and are still rare or have minimal representation in some medical schools and regions of the country. It stands to reason that with the lack of representation this far up the stream/pipeline to becoming a Hand surgeon, the chances of making it to becoming a surgery specialist such as a Hand surgeon are difficult but not impossible.

Although these disparities exist, it is possible to build a community and find supportive mentorship in medical school. Organizations such as the J. Robert Gladden Orthopedic Society (JRGOS), Nth Dimensions, Ruth Jackson Foundation, The Perry Initiative, American Society for Plastic Surgery Recruitment of Accomplished and Diverse Medical-student Applicants into Plastic Surgery, Student National Medical Association, Latino Medical Student Association, and Asian Pacific American Medical Student Association are student organizations that are incredibly useful in building a network.

During medical school, it is important to build a network and a record of experiences that make you a good candidate for your chosen residency. Aspects to consider include clinical experiences, basic science or clinical research, and leadership participation. Resources that can help with gathering these experiences are the network organizations previously mentioned and also scholarship opportunities that are dedicated to diversity, equity, and inclusion (DEI) initiatives. The importance

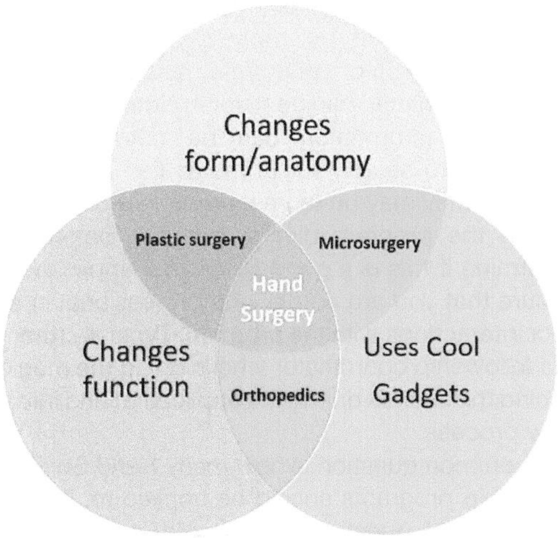

Fig. 1. Hand surgery is a special surgical subspeciality. It includes changing form/anatomy, function, and the use of technology. These principles are common in orthopedic surgery, Plastic Surgery, and microsurgery. Combined these skills make a great Hand surgeon.

of identifying mentorship and sponsorship becomes vital for the success of any medical student pursing a competitive field.

To improve the chances of matching for residency, it becomes critically important to seek mentors/sponsors and build a network. Shadowing is the best way a mentor that fits the individual well. If you are unable to find a mentor at your institution, consider searching for mentorship at other institutions if needed. Spending time with attending physicians during their typical workday is important to deciding if this field is the correct fit for you. Research suggests that medical schools with a small number of UIM faculty in orthopedic surgery produce lower numbers of residents from a UIM background.[7] Remember that you likely will not find a mentor or sponsor at your institution who looks just like you; however, it always becomes worthwhile to find a supportive mentor. In addition, it is natural as a female student to find female mentorship, which may or may not be in your desired field. Always be diligent to find the next individual that you can add to your supportive team.

Social media has become very important in building networks especially for minority communities. Social media platforms such as Twitter, Instagram, Facebook, and TikTok are easily accessible and are powerful ways to learn about each individual medical school and also to learn about resources offered for medical school and residency/fellowship training. In addition, for those who may not have a Hand Surgery home program, this is another avenue to reach out to Hand surgeons directly for mentorship.

Research suggests that minority students have more difficulty seeking and receiving mentorship opportunities for research and also shadowing/clinical experiences.[5] It is important to create these networks to learn from and to take advantage of these opportunities. Other than an in-person audition rotation or sub-internship, residency selection is heavily based on previous experiences on a Curriculum Vitae. Please note that basic science and clinical research will be valued more than other experiences when applying for residency. In addition, all institutions are not created equal, and therefore, there will be a significant variability of research opportunities available that may require students to consider either performing research at another institution or taking a year to perform dedicated research at another institution. These decisions for dedicated time to perform research should be closely guided by a trusted mentor who helps navigate the student through the competitiveness of the specialty.

With the recent change of Step 1 of the board test series becoming pass/fail, testing will hopefully be less emphasized in the selection of residency candidates; however, there will always be screening measures taken (ie, Step 2). Standardized testing is difficult, and it is worthwhile to seek resources to ensure that you have time to study to pass these tests without undue issues. Your goal in medical school is to match into a residency program that has a strong Hand Surgery program if possible. This will afford opportunities to further develop your interest in Hand Surgery and help you with making the process for applying easier given more opportunities for research and mentorship.

Residency: Explore Hand Surgery

Residency training in orthopedic and Plastic Surgery have wide spectrum of experiences within this subspecialized field. Although hand call can be a good way to experience Hand Surgery, one should understand that fingertip injuries and hand infections are only a small part of a career in Hand Surgery. Besides these standard rotations that you have within your residency, it is advisable to look at the operating room (OR) schedule of the Hand Surgery service to find interesting cases to observe. In addition, there are typically Hand Surgery conferences that occur on a weekly basis where didactics, clinical cases, and journal clubs would be another avenue to learn about the field and demonstrate interest by showing up engaged.

Residency serves as another barrier to becoming a Hand surgeon as a UIM applicant. In orthopedic, plastic, and general surgery, match rates among UIM applicants are lower than what is reported for medical student matriculates. There are also not many applicants from UIM backgrounds.[8,9] Similar to medical school, there are groups including the Garnes Society, the Latino/a Plastic Surgery Society, the Women of Color in PRS, the JRGOS, and the American Association of Latino Orthopedic Surgeons that provide resources, community, and mentorship/sponsorship for those from UIM backgrounds.

As with any surgery subspecialty, research and publications are one of the ways to differentiate your application from others. We all know that opportunities are unequal at each institution depending on resources, faculty, grants, and so forth. Despite these unequal opportunities, it is imperative that the resident remains assertive to enter this competitive field. This means meeting with as many Hand Surgery mentors and seeing if there is any potential for you to work on research projects. Be ready to commit to do a stellar job because getting a strong letter will distinguish one's application because the reputation of a strong mentor carries enormous influence to leaders in the field. Starting research projects early in residency, especially clinical projects allow you to finish these and get them published before applying into Hand Surgery. Another important aspect is to present this research at Hand Surgery specific meetings such as with the Hand Society (ASSH), the American Association for Hand Surgery, and any local hand society, for example, the New England Hand Society. Remember that Hand Surgery conferences are a great way to meet and make connections with other UIM Hand surgeons and Hand Surgery fellowship programs.

Hand Surgery Fellowship: Let the Differentiation Begin

Applying to Hand Surgery fellowships is really an extension of your training. Therefore, it becomes important to look at the training that you have had during your residency, speak with your mentors, attend hand meetings, meet current fellows, and identify a fellowship that you believe would offer additional training to make you a better and more complete Hand surgeon.

The ASSH provides a list of hand fellowships that can be applied to at www.assh.org/applications/s/fellowshipdirectory. It can be quite difficult to determine which programs an orthopedic or a Plastic surgeon can apply to. There is a combination of spots that are reserved for a specific type of applying resident. Most fellowship programs are equal opportunity and allow any resident within the fields of orthopedic, plastic, and general surgery to apply. Searching a Hand Surgery fellowship program's respective Web site for information can be helpful, although sometimes this information can be outdated and remember to search social media (ie, Instagram) because they may be represented there.[10,11] Contacting the program directly may be helpful to determine if this is a good fit for your application. Ensure that you are cordial and professional in all your interactions with the program. Typically, there is a fellowship coordinator who is doing the magic behind the scenes during the application and interview process.

A common question is how many Hand Surgery fellowship programs should be applied to. This is an individual question that should be reviewed with the program director at your institution or residency program director and will depend on the overall strength of your application. Most Plastic Surgery applicants apply to 10 to 20 programs; however, many orthopedic surgery residents may apply and interview at several more.[12] Gauging the number of programs to apply is based on how competitive your application is, guided by your mentors, and apply to as many as you feasibly can. Have a good story on why Hand Surgery is a good fit for you, this story you will communicate in your personal statement and interviews.

When considering Hand Surgery fellowships, it becomes important to consider several aspects that include clinic experience, operative experience, mentorship, rotation schedules, the number of fellows, the on-call requirements, didactic instruction, research opportunities, pediatric experience, geographic location, and so forth. An important consideration may be the amount of shoulder surgery that is performed within the fellowship which would most likely be not as relevant for a Plastic Surgery trained Hand Surgery Fellow. Similarly, a program that has a significant amount of replantation or microsurgery may be less relevant to an Orthopedic Surgery trained Hand Surgery Fellow who has accepted a future job with no plans to perform microvascular surgery. Hand fellowship programs may emphasize specific clinical areas of their respective fields including orthopedic and Plastic Surgery; however, having training in both aspects is what makes a strong Hand surgeon.[13] Our overall goal is to take the best possible care of patients and the more diverse the training the better. As Dr Quinn Capers IV, an interventional cardiologist and leader in diversity efforts, states "diversity drives excellence."

The disparity in representation is also present in fellowship programs. There also seems to be gender and racial preferences when choosing fellowship programs after residency training and orthopedic surgery.[14] Hand surgery was shown to be the most diverse subspecialty and fellowship program that was chosen after orthopedic surgery training. Unfortunately, this appearance of diversity is somewhat misleading given that African American, Latino/Hispanic, and Native American physicians continue to be underrepresented without much increase over the past few decades.

The Hand Surgery fellowship application is similar to applying to residency. The main difference is you will be in the trenches of your surgical residency when you are applying into fellowship. The application process starts your second to last year of residency, for example, in the fourth year of a 5-year orthopedic surgery residency or the fifth year of a 6-year Plastic Surgery residency. However, preparation for application starts several months earlier.

Recommendations While Applying for Fellowship

- Make sure to complete your application at the beginning of the application cycle.
- Plan ahead for the interview trail including vacation, call schedules, and so forth.
- Save up vacation time for interviews.
- Identify three to four letter writers for your letters of recommendation including the chief of your department, Hand Surgery fellowship directors, or research mentors. Make sure to meet with them and ask them to support your candidacy and give them at least 2 months warning to complete your letter.
- Talk to upper class women/men in your residency program that who applied in Hand Surgery; they may provide useful advice.
- Make sure to communicate with applicants who are also applying your year including your own residency or the other residency, whether orthopedic or Plastic Surgery applicants. You should be applying as colleagues rather than thinking of them as your competition. Make sure to use your colleagues as a resource while you are applying.

Once a resident has interviewed at multiple programs, the next step is the match process itself. The Hand Surgery Fellowship Match is administered by the National Resident Matching Program and occurs at the end of May of each year. This past year (2021) for appointment in 2022, the total programs were 91 for 187 available positions. It becomes incredibly exciting to finally be on your way to become a Hand surgeon as your defined career.

Identifying the "Right Fit" Training Programs

Identifying whether a residency or fellowship program is the "right fit" for the resident is an important consideration. The competitive nature of each step along the path to becoming a Hand surgeon includes medical school, residency, and fellowship programs are somewhat prohibitive when thinking or having the idea of a choice or being choosy when deciding where to go. For minority students, good training at a program that is supportive and is intentional about protecting and supporting their students from minority backgrounds is ideal. Identifying these programs can be difficult. The best way to do so or to reach out to mentors and current/past trainees from each program. The JRGOS also publishes a list of medical schools that trained the most African American Orthopedic surgeons.[15] The medical schools included are Howard, Meharry College, Harvard, and Morehouse.

A Life Interrupted for the Underrepresented in Medicine Individual

A challenge that is unique to students from a minority background is experiencing re-traumatization from world events such as the George Floyd's murder, the murder of Trayvon Martin, violence toward Asian Americans, and other horrific and very public displays of racial prejudice. Although this work was being written, another mass shooting targeting Black men and women occurred in Buffalo, NY. It is in these times where students may think the most alone in training programs that are predominantly White.

Although these national or worldwide events cannot be ignored or eliminated, it is the authors' belief that medical training programs, at each level of training, must support their trainees who may be emotionally or mentally affected by these incidents. In an effort for inclusivity, training programs must acknowledge these incidents and demonstrate their support for their staff and trainees through tangible actions. Providing trainees with mental health resources or simply breaks from training to cope with these events if necessary. Although it is difficult to identify which programs are supportive of their students from minority backgrounds, there are a few programs that stand out with their commitment to DEI. The Historically Black Colleges and Universities programs have been strong supporters for the advancement of minority students. Also, the University of Pennsylvania and Harvard are a few examples of universities that have been consistent supporters of diversity within their trainees.

SUMMARY

The perspective of the UIM Hand surgeon is valid. The hope is that this article can serve as an outline for those from atypical backgrounds to seek a career in Hand Surgery, despite the multiple obstacles. The authors are proud of their achievements to date, and the hope is that the readers will too be able to find a success pathway, with mentors and sponsor along the way, and reach their goal of becoming a well-trained Hand surgeon for every community.

REFERENCES

1. Earp BE, Mora AN, Rozental TD. Extending a Hand: Increasing Diversity at the American Society for Surgery of the Hand. J Hand Surg 2018;43(7):649–56. https://doi.org/10.1016/j.jhsa.2018.05.002.
2. Malhotra J, Rotter D, Tsui J, et al. Impact of Patient–Provider Race, Ethnicity, and Gender Concordance on Cancer Screening: Findings from Medical Expenditure Panel Survey. Cancer Epidemiol Biomarkers Prev 2017;26(12):1804–11. https://doi.org/10.1158/1055-9965.EPI-17-0660.
3. Greenwood BN, Carnahan S, Huang L. Patient–physician gender concordance and increased mortality among female heart attack patients. Proc Natl Acad Sci 2018;115(34):8569–74. https://doi.org/10.1073/pnas.1800097115.
4. Greenwood BN, Hardeman RR, Huang L, et al. Physician–patient racial concordance and disparities in birthing mortality for newborns. Proc Natl Acad Sci 2020;117(35):21194–200. https://doi.org/10.1073/pnas.1913405117.
5. Roberts SE, Shea JA, Sellers M, et al. Pursing a career in academic surgery among African American medical students. Am J Surg 2020;219(4):598–603. https://doi.org/10.1016/j.amjsurg.2019.08.009.
6. Lett E, Murdock HM, WU Orji, et al. Trends in Racial/Ethnic Representation Among US Medical Students. JAMA Netw Open 2019;2(9):e1910490. https://doi.org/10.1001/jamanetworkopen.2019.10490.
7. Okike K, Utuk ME, White AA. Racial and Ethnic Diversity in Orthopaedic Surgery Residency Programs. J Bone Jt Surg 2011;93(18):e107. https://doi.org/10.2106/JBJS.K.00108.
8. Keshinro A, Butler P, Fayanju O, et al. Examination of Intersectionality and the Pipeline for Black Academic Surgeons. JAMA Surg 2022;157(4):327. https://doi.org/10.1001/jamasurg.2021.7430.
9. Day CS, Lage DE, Ahn CS. Diversity Based on Race, Ethnicity, and Sex Between Academic Orthopaedic Surgery and Other Specialties: A Comparative Study. J Bone Jt Surg 2010;92(13):2328–35. https://doi.org/10.2106/JBJS.I.01482.
10. Silvestre J, Guzman JZ, Abbatematteo JM, et al. Evaluation of Content and Accessibility of Hand Fellowship Websites. HAND 2015;10(3):516–21. https://doi.org/10.1007/s11552-014-9732-9.
11. Trehan SK, Morrell NT, Akelman E. Accredited Hand Surgery Fellowship Web Sites: Analysis of Content and Accessibility. J Hand Surg 2015;40(4):778–82. https://doi.org/10.1016/j.jhsa.2015.01.024.
12. Meals C, Osterman M. The Hand Surgery Fellowship Application Process: Expectations, Logistics, and Costs. J Hand Surg 2015;40(4):783–9. https://doi.org/10.1016/j.jhsa.2014.12.041.
13. Sears ED, Larson BP, Chung KC. Program Director Opinions of Core Competencies in Hand Surgery Training: Analysis of Differences between Plastic and Orthopedic Surgery Accredited Programs. Plast Reconstr Surg 2013;131(3):582–90. https://doi.org/10.1097/PRS.0b013e31827c6f54.
14. Poon S, Kiridly D, Brown L, et al. Evaluation of Sex, Ethnic, and Racial Diversity Across US ACGME–Accredited Orthopedic Subspecialty Fellowship Programs. Orthopedics 2018;41(5):282–8. https://doi.org/10.3928/01477447-20180828-03.
15. Nsekpong TB, Ode G, Purcell K, et al. A track record of diversity: Medical schools ranked by successful black applicants to orthopaedic residencies. J Natl Med Assoc 2022;114(2):156–66. https://doi.org/10.1016/j.jnma.2021.12.013.

LGBTQ+ Perspective in Hand Surgery

Surgeon and Patient

Joseph Paul Letzelter, MD[a,*], Julie Balch Samora, MD, PhD, MPH, FAAOS, FAOA[b]

KEYWORDS

• LGBTQT • Transgender • Gay • Lesbian • Hand feminization • Ally

KEY POINTS

- There is a lack of LGBTQ+ representation within Hand Surgery.
- LGBTQ+ patients and physicians face discrimination within the hospital and other medical environments.
- LGBTQ+ patients have needs that can be different from those of other patients.
- Understanding desires from the transitioning patient or transgender patient can help hand surgeons better serve their community.

INTRODUCTION

Lesbian, gay, bisexual, transgender, queer, and other sexual and gender minority (LGBTQ+) individuals face high levels of harassment and discrimination at work.[1,2] This discrimination negatively impacts their health, wages, job opportunities, workplace productivity, and job satisfaction. Twenty seven percent of LGBTQ+ individuals stated that they faced discrimination in the workplace due to their sexual orientation. Further 7% of LGBTQ individuals reported being fired due to their sexual orientation.[2] In 2020, approximately 5.6% of the US population identified as LGBTQ.[3] Interestingly, this figure is higher in younger generations with 20% of Generation Z and 10% of millennials openly identifying as LGBTQ+.[4] With the increasing percentage of the younger population identifying as LGBTQ+, more individuals from this group will be presenting as patients in Hand Surgery clinics and entering the medical field. At present, there is a lack of guidance for LGBTQ+ medical students and residents entering the field of Hand Surgery as well as knowledge to appropriately treat LGBTQ+ patients with musculoskeletal concerns. As a specialty, we have a unique ability to advocate for the LGBTQ+ community to make Hand Surgery a welcoming specialty for medical students, residents, attendings, and faculty, and importantly our patients.

Lack of Diversity in Hand Surgery

The lack of racial and gender diversity within Orthopedic Surgery has been well documented. According to the American Academy of Orthopaedic Surgeons (AAOS) Census, only 6% of practicing orthopedic surgeons are women, 2.2% are Hispanic, and 2% are black.[5–7] Although no study has yet investigated the proportion of practicing orthopedic surgeons who identify as LGBTQ+, only 1.8% of LGBTQ+ students are entering the field of Orthopedic Surgery, which is lower than all other specialties.[8] A study of 63,721 graduating medical students found that 6.3% identified as LGBTQ+.[9] Sitkin and Pachankis[10] found that sexual and gender minorities (SGM) tend to shy away from competitive specialties, with the percentage of SGM in each specialty being inversely related to

[a] Orthopaedic Surgery Department, Children's National Medical Center, 111 Michigan Avenue Northwest, West Wing 1.5, Washington, DC 20010, USA; [b] Orthopaedic Surgery, Nationwide Children's Hospital, 700 Children's Drive; T2E-A2700, Columbus, OH 43205, USA
* Corresponding author. 50 V Street, Northwest, Washington, DC 20001.
E-mail address: JPL34@georgetown.edu

Hand Clin 39 (2023) 79–86
https://doi.org/10.1016/j.hcl.2022.08.005

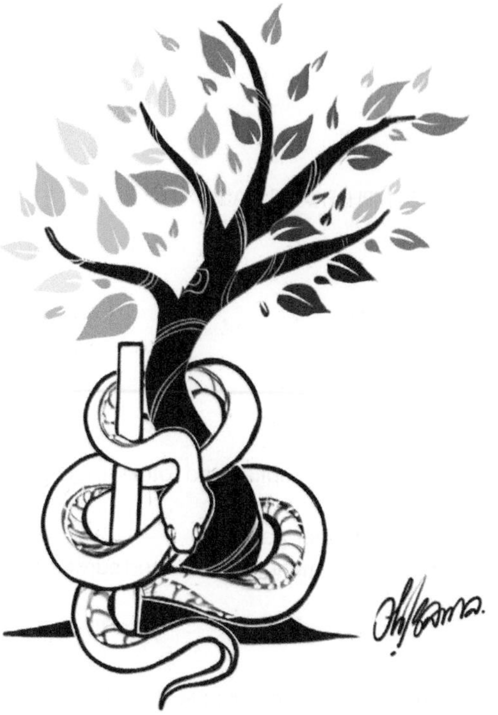

Fig. 1. Logo for Pride Ortho, an organization of LGBTQ+ individuals and their allies in Orthopedic Surgery. (*Courtesy of* Pride Ortho; with permission.)

specialty competitiveness. Furthermore, SGM students cite multiple factors that influence specialty choice, including personality fit, role models, specialty content, and work-life balance.

Students also report feeling there are cultural "in-groups" and "out-groups" when applying to a specific specialty. Gerull and colleagues[11] found students feeling in the "in-group" identified a sense of belonging in the field. The students' perceived stereotypes about Orthopedic Surgery included interest in sports, Caucasian race, male, heterosexual, dominant personality, and athletic physical build. Those who did not fit into those categories were more likely to feel part of the out-group. Those in the out-group reported their experiences within Orthopedic Surgery further reinforced their lack of identity alignment, furthered decreasing their interest in orthopedics.

The lack of LGBTQ+ medical students entering Orthopedic Surgery may be a detriment to the specialty, because we are not attracting the best and brightest. A study by Mittleman[12] found that gay men earn advanced degrees at higher rates than any other demographic group. About 6% of gay men in the United States have an advanced degree, which is 50% higher than heterosexual men. This figure holds true for gay men in the four largest racial/ethnic groups. An increasing proportion of advanced degree holders may identify as LGBTQ+ as a higher percentage of young adults in the general population identify as LGBTQ+.[13] Adults born between 1997 and 2003, considered Generation Z, identify as LGBTQ+ at a rate of 21%, which is double the percentage of millennials identifying as LGBTQ+. This observation likely indicates that an increasing number of the top students are likely to be LGBTQ+. It is timely for Orthopedic Surgery to create an inclusive environment to encourage the brightest into the specialty. LBGTQ+ medical students may be some of the most competitive students, but Orthopedic Surgery and thus Hand Surgery is missing out on these exceptional candidates due to perception and environment. The students with the most passion for a given field are the most likely to advance that field.

To encourage more LGBTQ+ students to pursue Hand Surgery, we need to recruit them at the medical student and residency level into Plastic Surgery, Orthopedic Surgery, and General Surgery. Pride Ortho is a nonprofit organization that was created to provide mentorship, networking, and a sense of belonging for LGBTQ+ members of the Orthopedic community (**Fig. 1**). By focusing on education and research, the organization aims to improve diversity and promote professional advancement of LGBTQ+ members of our community. To encourage more LGBTQ+ participation in Hand Surgery, we need to connect students/residents with mentors early on in their careers. We also need to increase national visibility of LGBTQ+ Plastic, Orthopedic, and General Surgeons, which demonstrates that LGBTQ+ trainees can thrive in practice as an LGBTQ+ hand surgeon.

Allyship

Once we are able to recruit students from the LGBTQ+ community, we have to understand how to support them. Being an ally has an immeasurable effect on not only the LGBTQ+ community within institutions, including surgeons, ancillary staff, patients, and caregivers. Being an ally in surgical specialties requires not only advocating for the LGBTQ+ community but also teaching others to be allies, and recruiting residents within the community.

A study by Heiderschiet and colleagues evaluated the experiences of LGBTQ+ General Surgery residents.[14] The investigators found 47.5% of LGBTQ+ residents experienced sexual harassment, 60% experienced discrimination, and 75% experienced bullying. These percentages were all significantly higher than their non-LGBTQ+ coresidents. LGBTQ+ residents were more likely to consider leaving their program and to consider suicide compared with their non-LGBTQ+ coresidents. When adjusting for mistreatment, LGBTQ+ residents had similar rates of consideration of suicide compared with the overall group. This indicates that mistreatment by attendings is one of the most common sources for suicidality among LGBTQ+ residents. Increasing visibility of allies and increasing the understanding of the importance of being an ally can minimize these numbers and enable trainees to feel seen, supported, and included.

Residents who have had training on LGBTQ+ allyship improve their objective ally scores as well as their openness and support of LGBTQ individuals[15]; this highlights the need for residencies and programs, especially ones in which the prevalence of LGBTQ+ patients is low, to create programs aimed at teaching faculty, residents, and students about the importance of being an ally. By creating an organization that is open and full of allies, one can create a group that continues to foster increased development and collaboration among both residents and faculty in a positive environment.

LGBTQ+ Physicians and Residents

Discrimination against LGBTQ+ physicians and patients has been an ongoing issue. A study by Schatz and O'Hanlan[16] demonstrated that many LGBTQ+ physicians experienced discrimination and witnessed discrimination against LGBTQ+ patients. This study, which was performed in 1994, found that 17% of respondees were denied privileges or promotions due to their sexual orientation. Thirty-four percent of respondees experienced some form of verbal harassment from a colleague.

A follow-up study by Eliason and colleagues[17] in 2011 found that 15% of respondees experienced harassment from a colleague; 34% witnessed discrimination against LGBTQ+ patients, and 65% had heard disparaging remarks about LGBTQ+ individuals. This mistreatment leads many LGBTQ+ physicians to feel less satisfied at work and results in lower rates of retention.[18] We need to work actively to create a welcoming environment for LGBTQ+ colleagues to continue to elevate the practice of Hand Surgery and improve care for all our patients.

It has been shown that underserved patients have better outcomes when treated by gender and ethnically diverse physicians.[19] Thus we should continue to recruit hand surgeons from diverse backgrounds. SGM trainees and physicians have experienced bias, discrimination, and harassment due to their sexual orientation or gender identity.[20] Among LGBTQ+ General Surgery residents, more than half reported hiding their sexual identity due to fears of mistreatment and discrimination.[21] By hiding their identity, these surgeons are less able to be who they are, which impacts their relationships with their colleagues and attendings. The inability to be oneself at work results in a negative feedback loop, with an inability to make connections with attendings, leading to a perception of being less competent, which can then lead to anxiety and a poorer performance.

LGBTQ+ Patients

Discrimination against LGBTQ+ individuals has been well documented. Human immunodeficiency virus has affected the gay male population more than any other population, which created a stigma within this cohort. Discrimination toward LGBTQ+ patients within the health care system has led many LGBTQ+ patients to be wary of this environment.[22,23] Many delay or avoid care altogether due to fear of being harassed, undermined, or not seen. Orthopedic Surgery is perceived as the least welcoming and inclusive specialty to SGM.[10] By understanding the specific needs and concerns of the LGBTQ+ population, we can change the culture within our specialties to make these patients feel more accepted and improve overall care.[24]

A key area for improvement is to address patients appropriately, with care not to misgender anyone, which requires treating everyone as if you are unassuming about their gender and pronouns. Electronic medical records should highlight preferred names and pronouns, which should be used. When seeing any patient, it is best to begin the conversation with "Who am I meeting today?" or "I am Dr So and so, what may I call you?" This puts patients at ease, especially those in the LGBTQ+ community who otherwise may have anxiety when seeing a health care provider. **Table 1** provides a list to help members of the hand community better understand terms.

Transgender Patients

More than 1 of every 200 people identify as transgender. Transgender is defined as an individual whose sex assigned at birth (usually based on external genitalia) does not align with one's gender identity (psychological sense of gender). The terms transgender, transexual, trans, gender incongruent, and genderqueer are adjectives for people with gender identities not aligned with

Table 1
Terms in LGBTQ+ nomenclature

Term	Definition
Ally	Someone who actively supports the LGBTQ+ community. This person can be straight and cisgendered or someone from within LGBTQ+ community supporting each other
Asexual	Someone who has a complete or partial lack of sexual attraction or lack of sexual interest. Asexual people exist on a spectrum and can range from no, minimal, or conditional sexual attraction
Bisexual	A person who is emotionally, sexually, or romantically attracted to individuals from more than one sex, gender, or gender identity
Cisgender	A term that is used to identify someone whose gender identity aligns with their sex at birth
Gay	An individual who is sexually attracted to someone of the same sex. Can include men, women, and nonbinary individuals
Gender binary	A system in which there are only 2 categories of male and female and those of each category are expected to align with their sex assigned at birth along with gender expressions and traditional roles
Gender identity	A person's innermost concept as male, female, both, or neither. This is how individuals perceive themselves and what they call themselves. This can be the same or different from their sex assigned at birth
Gender nonconforming	A person who behaves in a manner that does not align with the traditional expectations of their gender, or whose gender expression does not fit neatly into a category
Intersex	A person that is born with a variety of differences in their sex traits and reproductive anatomy
Lesbian	A woman who is attracted either emotionally, romantically, or sexually to another woman
Nonbinary	An adjective describing a person who does not identify exclusively as man or woman
Pansexual	A person who has the potential for emotional, romantic, or sexual attraction to people of any gender, although not necessarily simultaneously
Queer	A term used to express a spectrum of identities and orientations that are counter to mainstream
Sexual orientation	An inherent or immutable enduring emotional, romantic, or sexual attraction to other people. Sexual orientation is independent of sexual identity
Transgender	An umbrella term for people whose gender identity and/or expression is different from the cultural expectations based on the sex they were assigned at birth. This is independent of sexual orientation
Transitioning	A series of processes that some transgender people undergo to live more fully as their true gender

Data from Glossary of Terms (2021, May 30). Human Rights Campaign. Available at: https://www.hrc.org/resources/glossary-of-terms.

those they were assigned at birth. Transgender men have a male identity and were recorded as female at birth. Alternatively, transgender females were recorded as male at birth but have a female identity.

Many trans individuals may experience gender dysphoria. Gender dysphoria is the psychological distress an individual may feel when their sex assigned at birth does not match their gender identity. Gender dysphoria is a mental health diagnosis described in the *Diagnostic and Statistical Manual of Mental Disorders, 5th Edition*. Some transgender patients may pursue gender affirmation procedures to better align their physical appearance with their gender identity. The World Professional Association for Transgender Health provides guidelines for the surgical management of transgender patients. Before pursuing gender affirmation surgery, transgender patients must be in the care of a mental health professional who must document persistent gender dysphoria. Depending on the type of surgery, the patient may need to have taken 12 months of hormone therapy. Similarly, many commercial insurance companies in the United States require patients to have a diagnosis of gender dysphoria before undergoing gender-affirming procedures or treatments.[25]

Safer and Tangpricha[26] presented some key clinical points when caring for the transgender patient. No medical or procedural treatment is indicated before puberty. Once puberty starts there are medical (hormone) treatments to delay puberty and the development of secondary sex characteristics until a diagnosis of persistent gender dysphoria can be made. The most important consideration in the treatment of transgender patients is that every individual has unique goals when transitioning. Surgery and medical treatments should be tailored to each patient based on their interests and associated risks.

Ramsey and colleagues[27] conducted a study looking at the unique factors orthopedic surgeons should consider when caring for transgender patients. The investigators discussed issues that affect this population of patients including the role hormone therapy has on fracture risk and healing, perioperative infection, and venous thromboembolism. When treating someone transitioning, it is important to document if they are on hormone replacement therapy to stratify their risk for venothromboembolism, especially when performing a procedure.

Transitioning Procedures for the Transgender Patient

Hand feminization

Within the field of Hand Surgery, there are limited opportunities where we have the ability to assist individuals who are transitioning. One area where we can help is in hand feminization for transgender females. When many people think of transitioning, the most common procedures thought of are hormone replacement as well as procedures on the chest, face, and/or genitals. However, the hand is an area that is immediately visible to others and can be a cause of concern for many individuals transitioning.

Although gender affirmation of the hand is important to many patients, there is lack of research into this area. A study by Lee and colleagues[28] found that the female hand is approximately 25% smaller than the male hand. The masculine wrist is also proportionately wider than the female wrist. The ideal masculine hand appears slightly more square and muscular, whereas the feminine hand tends to be more slender.[29]

For the dorsum of the hand, desirable characteristics for a masculine hand include limited subcutaneous fat, whereas less prominent vasculature is more desirable for a feminine hand. The feminine hand is characterized by more subcutaneous fat and minimally noticeable tendons, unlike masculine hands.[29,30] When looking at the fingers and nails the ideal feminine hand has long, slender, hairless fingers. Nails also add to the feminization of fingers. Long nails add to the perception of long, slender, delicate fingers. Masculine nails tend to be short and square.[29]

Despite gender, many people favor a younger-appearing hand. A youthful hand has no wrinkles and supple skin. Aging predominantly affects the dorsum of the hand. The most common findings in an aging hand include wrinkles, dermal atrophy, bulging veins, and thickened joints.[31] Aging hands also show increased bony prominence due to loss of dorsal fat.[32] This increase in bony prominence along with the increase in size of the joints due to aging leads to the overall masculinization of the hand in all populations. For females transitioning to males, this is an overall benefit in terms of the hand looking more masculine. However, for transgender females, this is not ideal.

Surgical techniques

Most surgical techniques and therapies are aimed at feminization of the hand and increasing youthfulness of the hand. To date, there are no documented therapies for masculinization of the hand; however, as all hands age they do tend to appear more masculine. There is also no role for lengthening or shortening fingers due to the morbidity associated with the treatments.

Fat grafting

When feminizing a hand, one of the principles is to decrease the visibility of the underlying tendons and veins; this can be done with fat grafting, which can increase the smoothness of the dorsal hand. Donor sites are the abdomen, thigh, and flanks.[33,34] Fat grafting has generally high patient satisfaction results and a low risk profile. The most common complications of fat grafting include paresthesias, edema, hematoma, and ecchymoses.[33,34] One concerning complication for patients is some experience a difference in the absorption of the fat, which can cause irregular contours.[35]

Fat can also be injected into the lateral aspects of the fingers to treat fat wasting between the

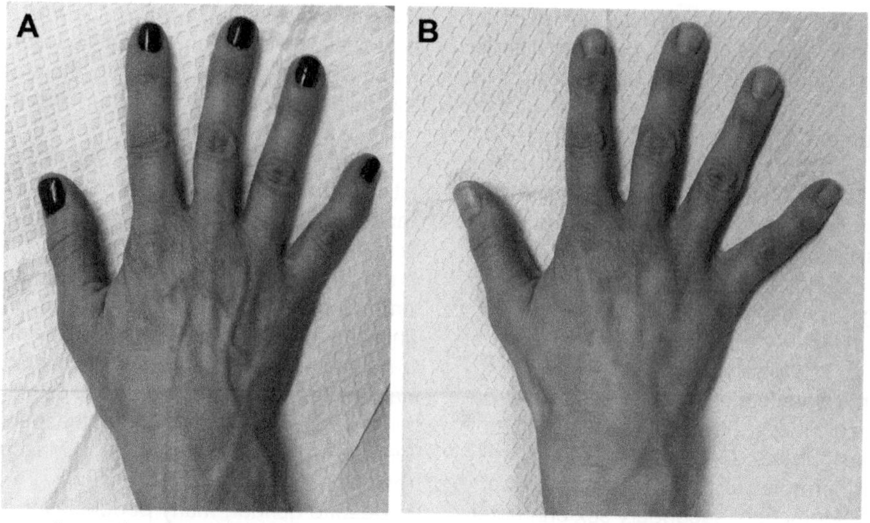

Fig. 2. Filler can be used to feminize the dorsum of the hand. (*A*) Preinjection with filler; (*B*) postinjection with filler shows the decrease in prominence of veins and increased smoothness of the dorsum of the hand. (*Courtesy of* Michael Somenek, MD, Washington, DC.)

joints. This procedure carries more risk, because the injections are closer to the neurovascular bundle, which can cause issues with vascularity to the digit as well as paresthesias and is thus not recommended.

Hand lift

The hand lift, also known as distal, dorsal superior extremity plasty, is performed by excising extra skin from the dorsum of the hand and wrist. The skin from the dorsum of the wrist is excised with minimal undermining to protect the draining venous architecture. This procedure is aimed at decreasing wrinkles, but does not affect the appearance of veins or tendons. The hand lift may help the dorsum of the hand appear smoother and thus more feminine.[36,37] Patient satisfaction is high, and risks include damage to branches of the radial and ulnar nerve, wound dehiscence, and decreased range of motion[36,38]; this can be a beneficial procedure for feminization, but it also leaves a scar and may be best done in concert with either fat grafting or filler to the dorsum of the hand.

Nonsurgical Techniques

Fillers

Injectable filler can be used to increase the volume in the dorsum of the hand not only to feminize the hand but also to increase the youthfulness of the hand appearance. Injectable filler can be used as an alternative to fat grafting, which decreases donor site morbidity (**Fig. 2**). Dermal grafts increase feminization by creating a smooth contour and decreasing visibility of the tendons and vascular structures; this is relatively safe with a similar complication profile as fat grafting. However, with fillers there is a possibility of developing a foreign body granuloma, which usually requires surgical excision or injection of steroids into the granuloma.[39]

Sclerotherapy

Sclerotherapy can also be used to decrease visibility of vasculature in the dorsum of the hand. The solution used is commonly sodium tetradecyl sulfate or pilodocanolis and is injected into the target vein. Common adverse effects include telangiectatic matting, ulcerations, hyperpigmentation, erythema, pruritis, and pain.[40]

Hormone therapy

Estrogen therapy increases body fat by 33% in the upper extremity in transgender women[41]; this results in an increase of body fat in the dorsum of the hand to help feminize the hand. Conversely, administering testosterone leads to an increase in lean muscle mass and decreases subcutaneous fat thus masculinizing the hand.

Hair removal

Many trans females desire the removal of body hair. Specifically, the dorsum of the hand tends to have more hair in a masculine hand compared with a feminine hand. Electrolysis, laser hair removal, and intense pulse light can all be used to decrease and remove hair. Electrolysis involves inserting a needle into the hair follicle and permanently removes the hair. Laser hair removal and intense pulse light source remove hair by damaging the follicular bulb, but leave the follicle intact; this leads to decreased and finer hair.

Laser and light therapy

Laser and light therapy can help target signs of photoaging including wrinkles. These therapies can help remove sunspots, which is neither feminizing nor masculinizing, but instead adds to the youthfulness of the hand's appearance. Nonablative fractional lasers penetrate into the dermis and stimulate neocollagenesis, which improves skin texture.[42] Intense pulse light produces dermal heating, which induces collagen production in the dermis; this improves fine skin wrinkles and increases smoothness of the hand.[43]

SUMMARY

An increasing proportion of the population is identifying as LGBTQ+. As leaders in our field, we must create and maintain a welcoming, open, and inclusive environment for everyone, from medical students, to patients, support staff, and partners. By creating an inclusive environment, we stand to attract some of the best applicants into the field of Hand Surgery. We must improve care for our LGBTQ+ patients, which includes being open to how they identify, treating them with respect, and trying to understand what treatment and care they are seeking.

CLINICS CARE POINTS

- Sexual and gender minorities tend to shy away from prestigious specialties including Orthopedic and Plastic Surgery.
- An increasing proportion of advanced degree holders identify as LGBTQ+ as a higher percentage of young adults in the general population identify as LGBTQ+.
- Residents who have had training on LGBTQ+ allyship improve objective ally scores as well as their openness and support of LGBTQ individuals.
- By increasing awareness and inclusivity, the field of Hand Surgery stands to possibly recruit top medical students from a diverse background.
- Treating a transgender patient requires openness in understanding the unique requests and needs they have, including a range of treatments for feminization of the hand.

DISCLOSURE

The authors have nothing to disclose.

REFERENCES

1. James SE, Herman JL, Rankin S, et al. The report of the 2015 US transgender survey. Washington, DC: National Center for Transgender Equality; 2016.
2. Sears B, Mallory C. Documented evidence of employment discrimination & its effects on LGBT people. Los Angeles, CA: The Williams Institute, UCLA School of Law; 2011.
3. Jones JM. LGBT identification rises to 5.6%in latestU.S. estimate. https://news.gallup.com/poll/329708/lgbt-identification-rises-latest-estimate.aspx. [Accessed 24 February 2022].
4. GLAAD. Accelerating Acceptance. 2017. Available at: https://www.glaad.org/files/aa/2017_GLAAD_Accelerating_Acceptance.pdf.
5. Bennett CL, Baker O, Rangel EL, et al. The gender gap in surgical residencies. JAMA Surg 2000; 155(9):893–4.
6. Van Heest AE, Agel J, Samora JB. A 15-Year Report on the Uneven Distribution of Women in Orthopaedic Surgery Residency Training Programs in the United States. JB JS Open Access 2021;6(2):e200015.
7. International Orthopaedic Diversity Alliance. Diversity in orthopaedics and traumatology: a global perspective. EFORT Open Rev 2020;5(10):743–52.
8. American Academy of Orthopaedic Surgeons. Orthopaedic Practice in the U.S. 2018. 2018. https://www.aaos.org/globalassets/quality-and-practice-resources/census/2018-census.pdf.
9. Mori WS, Gao Y, Linos E, et al. Sexual Orientation Diversity and Specialty Choice Among Graduating Allopathic Medical Students in the United States. JAMA Netw Open 2021;4(9):e2126983. PMID: 34591110.
10. Sitkin NA, Pachankis JE. Specialty Choice Among Sexual and Gender Minorities in Medicine: The Role of Specialty Prestige, Perceived Inclusion, and Medical School Climate. LGBT Health 2016; 3(6):451–60.
11. Gerull KM, Parameswaran P, Jeffe DB, et al. Does Medical Students' Sense of Belonging Affect Their Interest in Orthopaedic Surgery Careers? A Qualitative Investigation. Clin Orthop Relat Res 2021; 479(10):2239–52.
12. Mittleman Joel. Intersecting the Academic Gender Gap: The Education of Lesbian, Gay and Bisexual America. SocArXiv 2021.
13. Source: CNN. https://www.cnn.com/2022/02/17/us/lgbtq-population-increase-gallup-cec/index.html. [Accessed 24 February 2022].
14. Heiderscheit EA, Schlick CJR, Ellis RJ, et al. Experiences of LGBTQ+ Residents in US General Surgery

Training Programs. JAMA Surg 2022;157(1):23–32. https://doi.org/10.1001/jamasurg.2021.5246. PMID: 34668969; PMCID: PMC8529519.
15. Grova MM, Donohue SJ, Bahnson M, et al. Allyship in Surgical Residents: Evidence for LGBTQ Competency Training in Surgical Education. J Surg Res 2021;260:169–76. Epub 2020 Dec 17. PMID: 33341680.
16. Schatz B, O'Hanlan K. Anti-gay discrimination in medicine: results of a national survey of lesbian, gay and bisexual physicians: American Association of Physicians for Human Rights. San Francisco, CA: AAPHR); 1994.
17. Eliason MJ, Dibble SL, Robertson PA. Lesbian, gay, bisexual, and transgender (LGBT) physicians' experiences in the workplace. J Homosex 2011;58: 1355–71.
18. Patridge EV, Barthelemy R, Rankin SR. Factors impacting the academic climate for LGBQ STEM faculty. J Women Minorities Sci Eng 2014;20.
19. Gomez LE, Bernet P. Diversity improves performance and outcomes. J Natl Med Assoc 2019; 111:383–92.
20. Przedworski JM, Dovidio JF, Hardeman RR, et al. A Comparison of the Mental Health and Well-Being of Sexual Minority and Heterosexual First-Year Medical Students: A Report From the Medical Student CHANGE Study. Acad Med 2015;90:652–9.
21. Lee KP, Kelz RR, Dubé B, et al. Attitude and perceptions of the other underrepresented minority in surgery. J Surg Educ 2014;71:e47–52.
22. Legal L. When health care isn't caring: lambda Legal's survey of discrimination against LGBT people and people with HIV. New York: Lambda Legal; 2010. p. 1–26.
23. Tjepkema M. Health care use among gay, lesbian and bisexual Canadians. Health Rep 2008;19: 53–64.
24. Chu A, Lin JS, Moontasri NJ, et al. LGBTQ+ in Orthopaedics: Creating an Open and Inclusive Environment. J Am Acad Orthop Surg 2022;30(13): 599–606.
25. Accessing coverage for transition-related health care. New York: Lambda Legal. Available at: https://www.lambdalegal.org/know-your-rights/article/trans-health-care.
26. Safer J, Tangpricha V. Care of Transgender Persons. N Engl J Med 2019;381(25):2451–60.
27. Ramsey DC, Lawson MM, Stuart A, et al. Orthopaedic Care of the Transgender Patient. J Bone Joint Surg Am 2021;103:274–81.
28. Lee J, Nolan IT, Swanson M, et al. A Review of Hand Feminization and Masculinization Techniques in Gender Affirming Therapy. Aesthet Plast Surg 2021; 45(2):589–601. Epub 2020 Sep 30. PMID: 32997239.
29. Jakubietz RG, et al. Defining the basic aesthetics of the hand. Aesthet Plast Surg 2005;29(6):546–51.
30. Kos'cin'ski K. Hand attractiveness—its determinants and associations with facial attractiveness. Behav Ecol 2011;23(2):334–42.
31. Bains RD, Thorpe H, Southern S. Hand aging: patients' opinions. Plast Reconstr Surg 2006;117(7): 2212–8.
32. Hoevenaren IA, et al. Three-dimensional soft tissue analysis of the hand: a novel method to investigate effects of acromegaly. Eur J Plast Surg 2016;39(6): 429–34.
33. Agostini T, Perello R. Lipomodeling: an innovative approach to global volumetric rejuvenation of the hand. Aesthet Surg J 2015;35(6):708–14.
34. Fantozzi F. Hand rejuvenation with fat grafting: a 12-year single-surgeon experience. Eur J Plast Surg 2017;40(5):457–64.
35. Yun-Nan L, et al. Micro-autologous fat transplantation for rejuvenation of the dorsal surface of the aging hand. J Plast Reconstr Aesthet Surg 2018;71(4): 573–84.
36. Wendt JR. Distal, dorsal superior extremity plasty. Plast Reconstr Surg 2000;106(1):210–3.
37. Pozner JN, DiBernardo BE. Commentary on: minimal-scar handlift: a new surgical approach. Aesthet Surg J 2011;31(8):963–5.
38. Handle M, et al. Minimal-scar handlift: a new surgical approach. Aesthet Surg J 2011;31(8):953–62.
39. Park TH, et al. Clinical experience with complications of hand rejuvenation. J Plast Reconstr Aesthet Surg 2012;65(12):1627–31.
40. Fabi SG, Goldman MP. Hand rejuvenation: a review and our experience. Dermatol Surg 2012;38(7 Pt 2): 1112–27.
41. Klaver M, et al. Changes in regional body fat, lean body mass and body shape in trans persons using cross-sex hormonal therapy: results from a multicenter prospective study. Eur J Endocrinol 2018; 178(2):163–71.
42. Archer KA, Carniol P. Diode laser and fractional laser innovations. Facial Plast Surg 2019;35(3):248–55.
43. Goldberg DJ. New collagen formation after dermal remodeling with an intense pulsed light source. J Cutan Laser Ther 2000;2(2):59–61.

The International Medical Graduate Perspective in Hand Surgery

Legacy and Future Challenges

Uzair Qazi, MD[a], Laxminarayan Bhandari, MCh[b,*]

KEYWORDS

• International medical graduates • Legacy • Education

KEY POINTS

- International Medical graduates (IMGs) are an integral part of the United States health-care system and flagbearers of diversity.
- IMGs have contributed significantly to Hand Surgery in terms of skillsets, innovation, leadership, mentorship, and research.
- Numerous challenges exist for IMGs to successfully establish their practice in the United States.

Most International Medical Graduates (IMGs) are first-generation immigrants who plant the seeds of diversity not only in the health-care sector but also in the society at large. The contributions of IMGs to diversity are enormous. IMG physicians become the flag bearers of their countries in the United States, which is the "melting pot" of cultures and diversity. A patient visiting an IMG physician experiences a different accent, appearance, and culture. This broadens the perspective of the society, and encourages tolerance, understanding, and respect.

The American Academy of Family Physicians defines an IMG as a physician who received a basic medical degree from a medical school located outside the United States and Canada that is not accredited by a US accrediting body, the Liaison Committee on Medical Education (LCME), or the American Osteopathic Association.[1] IMGs enter the United States medical education system at different levels of training. They not only empower the system by plugging in gaps of physician shortages but also bring along inherent diversity.

However, not all IMGs are foreign nationals. American nationals who pursue their medical training abroad are also considered IMGs. Such students choose to train in a foreign country such as the ones in the Caribbean, Europe, or Asia for a multitude of reasons. Lower cost of education, exposure to different cultures, and training in international medicine are the main drivers.[2] Once they complete their medical education, they are also considered an IMG.

The 2 pathways for IMGs are (1) fresh IMG pursuing residency training in the United States or (2) specialist IMG pursuing fellowship training in the United States.

JOURNEY OF FRESH INTERNATIONAL MEDICAL GRADUATE GETTING INTO US RESIDENCY AND THEN FELLOWSHIP

A fresh IMG is someone who recently graduated from a medical school abroad. After completing medical school in a foreign country for 4 to 5 years and passing the United States Medical Licensing

[a] Division of Plastic/Reconstructive and Hand Surgery/Burn Surgery, Department of Surgery, University of Cincinnati College of Medicine, 231 Albert Sabin Way Suite MSB 2360A, Cincinnati, OH 45267, USA; [b] Kleinert Kutz Associates, 225 Abraham Flexner Way, Suite 700, Louisville, KY 40202, USA
* Corresponding author:
E-mail address: lax321@gmail.com

Hand Clin 39 (2023) 87–93
https://doi.org/10.1016/j.hcl.2022.08.006

Examinations, IMGs then apply for residency along with US seniors. This is followed by a lengthy process of multiple interviews culminating toward match day. The coveted residency positions are highly competitive, and it is not uncommon for IMGs to spend a year or two in research or preliminary positions to make themselves worthy of consideration. The competition to be invited for a residency interview is very fierce.

As per National Resident Matching Program (NRMP), about 5048 American IMGs applied for NRMP in 2022, of which only 3099 (or 61.4%) matched. For foreign IMGs, the number has declined further down to 58%. This is in stark contrast to US seniors with 93% matching into a residency position.[3] The situation gets worse in surgical specialties for IMGs. Of the 1619 categorical General Surgery positions, 1457 were given to American seniors and graduates, 80 to American IMGs and 81 to foreign IMGs. As expected, the IMGs fare worse in securing Orthopedic and Plastic Surgery positions, with 19/875 Orthopedic and 11/194 integrated Plastic Surgery positions going to IMGs.[3]

Many IMGs end up completing multiple years of preliminary positions in hopes of matching into a categorical position. Once successful in securing a categorical position, the residents take 5 to 6 years to complete their residency. Following residency, these IMG will be board-eligible in their respective specialty and can pursue either fellowship or employment opportunities within the United States. Candidates interested in Hand Surgery apply for the Hand Surgery match hosted by the American Society for Surgery of the Hand (ASSH). There are 97 fellowship programs accepting candidates from Orthopedic, Plastic, and General Surgery backgrounds.

Specialist International Medical Graduate Pursuing Fellowship Training in the United States

Less common are IMGs who enter the US training system after completing their residency in a foreign country. These IMGs are specialists in their basic specialties and come to the United States for further training, usually for fellowship training. Although some fellowship programs are more open to international candidates, most are not. In the Hand Surgery fellowship match 2021, of the 181 positions through the Hand Surgery match, 174 went to United States and Canadian graduates, 6 to American IMGs and 1 to a foreign IMG.[4]

To be eligible for an Accreditation Council for Graduate Medical Education (ACGME) accredited training position, The ACGME requires completion of an ACGME-accredited residency program, an AOA-approved residency program, a program with ACGME International Advanced Specialty Accreditation, or a Royal College of Physicians and Surgeons of Canada accredited, or College of Family Physicians of Canada accredited residency program located in Canada.[5] As most specialist IMGs are not trained from these programs, they do not qualify for an ACGME-accredited position. On rare occasion, the review committees for Orthopedic Surgery and Plastic Surgery can allow certain exceptions to the fellowship eligibility requirements for certain outstandingly qualified IMG applicants. Applicants accepted through this exception must have an evaluation of their performance by the Clinical Competency Committee within 12 weeks of matriculation.[5]

Foreign IMGs can obtain fellowship training in positions without ACGME accreditation. In Hand Surgery, the Christine M. Kleinert Institute has a parallel international program where 6 to 8 IMGs are trained annually. This program attracts fellows from all over the world. During the past 62 years, about 1300 fellows have been trained from 58 different countries.[6]

The fellowship training does not make the specialist IMG eligible to take US boards or the Subspeciality Certificate in Surgery of the Hand. Thus, they pursue one of the following pathways:

1. Return to their home country—Most IMGs return to their home country after completing their advanced training in the United States. Many such US fellowship-trained Hand surgeons have gone on to become world leaders in Hand Surgery and have started their own centers of excellence and fellowship programs, Ganga Hospital in Coimbatore, India being one such institute that attracts Hand surgeons from all over the world.[7]
2. Pursue further fellowships—Some IMGs continue seeking further training and advancing their skill set by pursuing fellowships in subspecialities of Orthopedic or Plastic Surgery.
3. Start working—Rarely are IMGs able to serve patients in their capacity as specialist Hand surgeons. As these IMGs are not board eligible, they face multiple challenges in licensing and credentialing as discussed later.
4. Pursue residency—Sometimes, following fellowship, the IMGs redo their residency in a basic specialty in the United States to be board-eligible. These fellows must compete with recent medical graduates to get into a residency position and restart their residency from the intern level, both very challenging and grueling circumstances.

LEGACY

Despite these hardships and hurdles, many IMGs have been very successful in their career as Hand surgeons in the United States and have contributed tremendously to this field. From being Society presidents to innovators, to teachers, IMGs have made the field of Hand Surgery very rich. The authors acknowledge the struggles and contributions of all IMGs through this article; however, due to space and time constraints, we briefly highlight a few cherry-picked contributors and their contributions. A comprehensive list of IMGs and their achievements, although essential, is a daunting task. The authors wholeheartedly acknowledge this criticism.

Skillset—Dr Tsu-min Tsai, Taiwan

When Joseph Kutz attended a meeting in Japan in 1974, he saw a young microsurgeon presenting a unique case of a 4-finger replant. What made the case unique was the fact that these fingers were previously replanted a few years ago. The patient suffered amputations of the same fingers again and this microsurgeon replanted them back—a feat never achieved before! This surgeon was Tsu-min Tsai. Impressed by his microsurgery skills and determination, Harold Kleinert and Hiram Polk, the chair of surgery at University of Louisville at that time, invited him to Louisville. During his visit, Dr Tsai demonstrated a successful replantation of a ring avulsion injury considered nonsalvageable by many at that time. Realizing the need to have such a skill set in the practice, Kleinert and Kutz asked Dr Tsai to join their group.

Bringing in such a skill set translated into clinical success. The survival rate of replants increased from the prevailing 40% to 90%. A triumph Dr Tsai is "most proud of" in his professional career spanning half a century. Worth mentioning here are 2 beneficiaries of Dr Tsai's amazing skills; the first man to walk on the moon and the man who got the most successful hand transplant to date (**Fig. 1**).

Even though he is now retired, Dr Tsai continues to participate actively in teaching the fellows. His teachings go beyond medicine, and he shares the secret of his success in these words—"Never be lazy for learning, avoid bad habits and keep good health."

Innovation: Dr Luis Scheker, Dominican Republic

"The need to solve problems leads to innovation," says Dr Luis Scheker who has described many innovative techniques, designed a prosthetic device that bears his name, and currently owns the company that manufactures this device (**Fig. 2**). Dr Luis Scheker came to the United States in 1982 looking forward to spending a year in Louisville and to head back to the Dominican Republic as the first microvascular surgeon in the country. However, the "assembly line Hand Surgery" at Louisville attracted him to stay here. "People need a hand to do everything" says Dr Scheker "and that was the appeal" to switch from Craniofacial Surgery to Hand Surgery. With support from "Futuristic" Harold Kleinert, Robert Acland, and others, Dr Scheker made Louisville his home.

For a patient with carpometacarpal arthritis, to reconstruct the intermetacarpal ligament, he designed the half flexor carpi radialis technique. Similarly, distal radioulnar joint (DRUJ) pain was

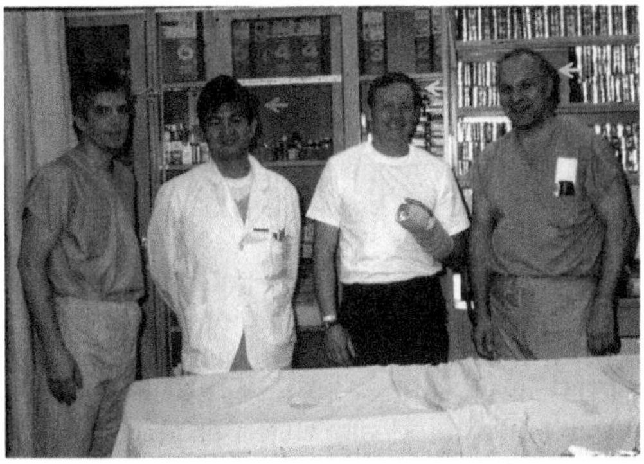

Fig. 1. Neil Armstrong (*green arrow*) with his replanted finger flanked by Dr Thomas Wolff (*red arrow*), Dr Tsu-min Tsai (*blue arrow*) on the right, and Dr Joseph Kutz (*yellow arrow*) on his left.

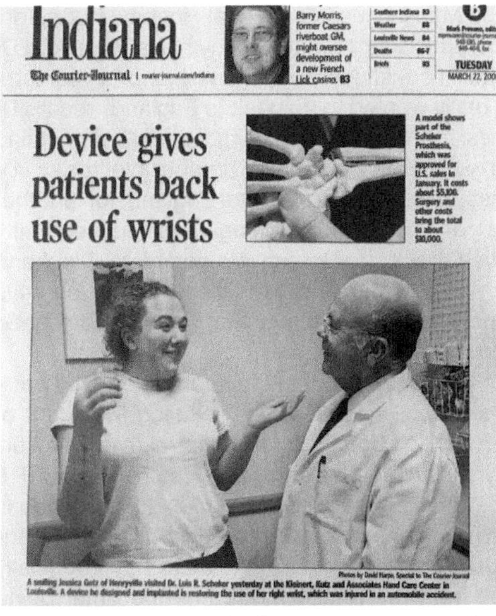

Indiana
The Courier-Journal
Barry Morris, former Caesars riverboat GM, might oversee development of a new French Lick casino. B3
TUESDAY
MARCH 22, 2005

Device gives patients back use of wrists

A model shows part of the Scheker Prosthesis, which was approved for U.S. sales in January. It costs about $5,100. Surgery and other costs bring the total to about $30,000.

Photos by David Harpe, Special to The Courier-Journal
A smiling Jessica Getz of Henryville visited Dr. Luis R. Scheker yesterday at the Kleinert, Kutz and Associates Hand Care Center in Louisville. A device he designed and implanted is restoring the use of her right wrist, which was injured in an automobile accident.

Fig. 2. Newspaper article showcasing Dr Luis Scheker, his prosthesis, and a patient happy with her result.

an unsolved problem at the time despite the moderate success of Darrach's procedure. In 1995, when encountered with a Vietnam veteran with a hand grenade explosion, Dr Scheker innovated a way to provide pronosupination. This innovation ultimately led to the birth of DRUJ prosthesis and the "rest is history."

Dr Scheker advises young IMGs looking for a career in Hand Surgery to find a suitable mentor, who would advise, give ideas, and even scrub in difficult cases. He recommends that a university setting would be ideally suited at the beginning of an IMG's career.

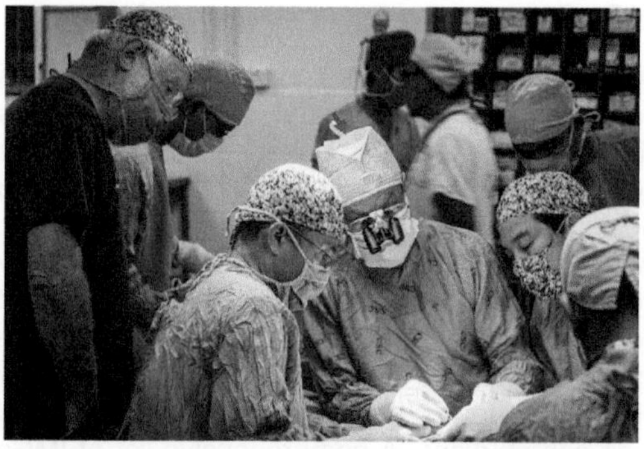

Fig. 3. Dr Neil Ford Jones (*red arrow*) teaching Hand Surgery to the local surgeons at Phnom Penh, Cambodia during one of the outreach programs.

Leadership: Dr Neil Jones, United Kingdom

Dr Jones's journey is as astonishing as it is unique, perhaps unparalleled. Under an exchange program between Oxford University and the Medical College of Wisconsin, Dr Jones was the first trainee to visit Milwaukee. What was supposed to be 1 year, turned out to be decades of serendipitous association between Dr Jones and American Hand Surgery.

"I had always wanted to go into one of the surgical specialties," says Dr Jones; however, Cardiac Surgery and Transplant Surgery seemed "mundane" and Neurosurgery "depressing." During his registrarship in Orthopedic Surgery, he found Hand Surgery "intriguing." Another fortuitous moment occurred, when he suddenly got a call from Dr William Grabb at the University of Michigan to join their residency program in Plastic Surgery. Following his residency, Dr Jones was selected for the Hand Surgery fellowship program at the Massachusetts General Hospital in Boston, under Dr Richard Smith. "In my naivety, I asked Dr Smith if I could delay the fellowship for a year later as I really wanted to go back to England" recalls Dr Jones, "fortunately, Dr Smith agreed"; something that would be considered impossible today. Dr Jones therefore returned to England for another year of fellowship training and subsequently moved back to Boston to complete his hand fellowship. These frequent transatlantic journeys earned him a reputation that he had "designed his own training program"!

Dr Jones has occupied multiple leadership positions in the United States, including President of the American Society for Reconstructive Microsurgery 2008 to 2009 and President of the ASSH 2015 to 2016. To put this in perspective, only 6 surgeons have ever been presidents of both these prestigious organizations and 2 of them have originally been from the United Kingdom—the other being Dr Graham Lister. During his presidency, Dr Jones promoted international collaboration (**Fig. 3**). He announced a new ASSH International Hand Surgery fellowship program, in which 3 young US Hand surgeons would spend 3 months operating in high volume Hand Surgery centers in China and India. He also developed the ASSH International Visiting Professor program in which a senior ASSH member visits several institutions in 2 developing countries to evaluate patients and teach Hand Surgery. Finally, he instructed the program chair of the annual ASSH meeting that all symposia and instructional courses should include at least one international Hand surgeon.[8]

Dr Jones's advice for aspiring leaders is to work their way up within an organization, developing a local, national, and international reputation. "Take part in committee activities and show yourself to be a good team player, organizer, and communicator" says Dr Jones, "Gather respect and you will advance in leadership."

Mentorship: Dr Milan Stevanovic, Serbia

> "The mediocre teacher tells. The good teacher explains. The superior teacher demonstrates. The great teacher inspires."—William Arthur Ward

Having mentored hundreds of medical students, residents, and fellows, Dr Milan Stevanovic has inspired many, who in turn have reached great heights making their mentor proud. Dr Stevanovic recalls one such event. While attending a talk on face transplants, Dr Stevanovic told the presenter how much he enjoyed the talk, the presenter, in turn, replied "Thank you for showing me the dissection techniques." To Dr Stevanovic's surprise, the presenter was a frequent attendee of his flap course and thus one of his students. Proudly recalling the meeting Dr Stevanovic says, "Teaching is an obligation. You teach and never know how much you influence."

Two factors influenced Dr Stevanovic's career. His math teacher and the Yugoslavian war. Being a math major, he wanted to pursue a career in electrical engineering emulating the Serbian legend, Nikola Tesla. However, his math teacher, who profoundly influenced him, directed him to take up medicine to help people. After completing his Orthopedic Surgery residency at the Medical University of Belgrade he entered the Joseph H. Boyes fellowship program, the oldest and most prestigious Hand Surgery fellowship of that time. He followed this with a microsurgery fellowship at Duke under Dr James R. Urbaniak. On his return to the University of Belgrade, he established the first microsurgery center with many firsts in the nation such as the first hand replant, toe transfer, free fibula, and so forth before the Yugoslavian civil war caused him to migrate back to the United States.

Back in the University of Southern California, Dr Stevanovic made multiple contributions such as chimeric medial thigh flap, increasing the survival of the medial skin on gracilis flap, emergency free functional muscle transfer, and has the unique distinction of performing 6-toe transfer in a single patient in 2 stages.

Dr Stevanovic (**Fig. 4**) advises the prospective IMGs to approach good mentors. "Good people like good people and where you are trained matters." For the prospective mentors, he advises that selecting the right candidates is most important, "it is like selecting the government." He prefers candidates with skills in sports/arts or literature because they have "a part of the brain that I don't have." "Respect the student and never be angry or suppress his/her ideas. Many times, these are better than your own."

Research: Dr Linda Cendales, Colombia

Research is an integral part of IMG's journey in establishing a career. One such passionate researcher who is contributing to the growth and innovation of Hand Surgery is Dr Linda Cendales.

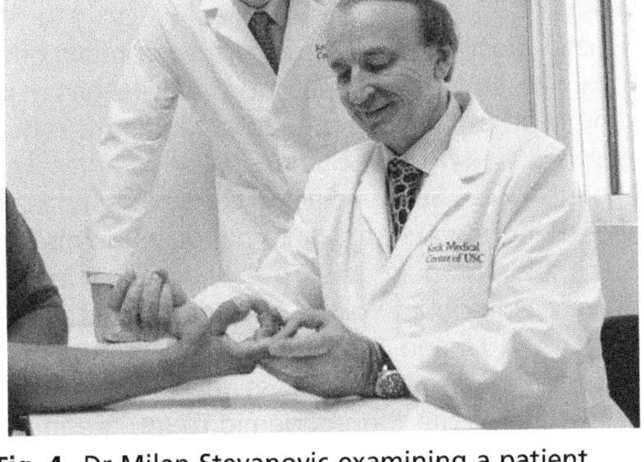

Fig. 4. Dr Milan Stevanovic examining a patient.

Dr Cendales is the only person in the United States to have completed formal fellowship training in both Hand and Microsurgery and Transplant Surgery. She finished her high school in Bogota, Colombia, her college in the Kingdom of Swaziland, and medical school in Mexico City, Mexico, where she opted to spend a year researching immunology and rheumatology at the National Institute of Medical Sciences.

What made her select this field? "Being passionate about one's interests is energizing" Dr Cendales recalls this passion when she encountered a woman in her 60s with severe rheumatoid arthritis. Immunosuppression was not as developed as it is today and despite being on multiple immunosuppressive medications, she had debilitating hand deformities. "What if we give her a hand transplant?.. she is already on immunosuppression and kidney transplants are performed routinely" reasoned Dr Cendales. However, it was a time when she "did not know or had spoken with anyone who had done a hand transplant."

"Once a challenge is identified, work hard to overcome it - by getting trained, working hard, and support from others." Moreover, this path led her to the Christine M. Kleinert Institute, where Dr Cendales spent 2 years with Dr Warren C. Breidenbach as the principal investigator and the rest of the team to establish the nation's first hand transplant program (**Fig. 5**).

Pursuing her passion, Dr Cendales became the first person to be accepted into the National Institute

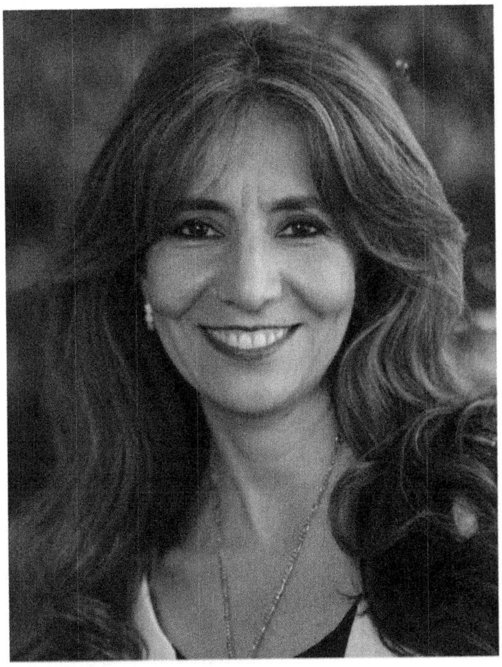

Fig. 5. Dr Linda Cendales.

of Health transplant and immunobiology fellowship where she established the primate model for vascularized composite tissue allotransplantation (VCA) that has the largest reported experience in the nonhuman primates VCA to date. She also established the currently accepted classification system for rejection of skin containing VCA. Dr Cendales went on to establish 2 more hand transplant programs one at Emory University in Georgia, Atlanta, and the other at Duke in North Carolina, where she currently heads the VCA program.

"There is no substitute for hard work" is the mantra Dr Cendales passes on to the next generation. Be "prudent, persistent, patient, and persevere. Do what you do well, and people will see it," says Dr Cendales "It is difficult to argue with a good result. Talent cannot be hidden."

Current and Future Challenges for International Medical Graduates

IMGs face a multitude of challenges. Visa and immigration issues are common hurdles and play a crucial role in career decisions. The decision to pursue a fellowship or a job, as well as the location of the job depends on the immigration status. Currently, most IMGs receive their training on a J-1 visa sponsored by the Educational Commission for Foreign Medical Graduates. Following training, to pursue a job in the United States, they need to obtain a J-1 waiver and subsequently an H1b visa. Not all prospective employers offer such waiver positions. These waiver positions are typically located in medically underserved areas, where the physicians must serve at least 3 years.[9] In addition, the H1b visa has a limitation of 7 years. To immigrate to the United States, the physician will need a green card. The process to obtain a green card can be long, especially for physicians from China and India.[10]

Another challenge for specialist IMGs is board certification. Although the IMGs who complete their residency in the United States are eligible to take their boards, those who enter through the fellowship pathway are not. Fellowship training does not allow candidates to receive board certification. Fortunately, The American Board of Plastic Surgery (ABPS), The American Board of Orthopedic Surgery (ABOS) as well as The American Board of Surgery (ABS) each have alternate pathways for board certification through an academic route.

The ABPS requires the specialist IMG to work in a division/department of Plastic Surgery that is ACGME–approved for a Plastic Surgery residency training program, as an Assistant or Associate Professor, for 7 consecutive years while being engaged in the teaching and training of Plastic Surgery residents. After attaining Associate Professorship and fulfilling several other criteria, the IMG can be deemed eligible to take the boards, contingent on the board's decision.[11] The ABOS pathway is open for Orthopedic surgeons who have independently practiced for at least 5 years in the United States while serving on the full-time academic teaching faculty in a single ACGME-accredited Orthopedic Surgery residency program.[12] Similarly, The ABS requires that the IMG must be employed as a full-time teaching faculty member at a LCME-accredited medical school and at an institution with an ACGME-accredited General Surgery residency training program. The accreditation of both the medical school and training program must span the 5 continuous years of employment.[13]

A third challenge is to get a state license, which is a prerequisite to working and fulfilling the above requirements. The license to practice is issued by respective state boards and this can also be a challenge for the specialist IMG due to the lack of ACGME-accredited training. The application process varies depending on the state.[14] It requires submission of all training materials, and frequently needs a prospective job offer and a personal appearance before the state licensing board. Often, IMGs can only obtain a limited institutional license to commence their job before subsequently getting a full unrestricted license.

In addition, even after getting a license and board certification, the fellowship-trained specialist IMG still may not be eligible to obtain the Subspecialty Certificate in Surgery of the Hand (previously known as CAQ hand). This is because, to be eligible for the Subspecialty certificate, the specialist IMG must have completed their fellowship in an ACGME-accredited position. If the fellowship was done in a nonaccredited position, the IMG is not eligible for the Subspecialty certificate. As previously discussed, not all Hand Surgery fellowship positions are ACGME-accredited positions. Even if an IMG completes an ACGME-accredited fellowship, the individual still needs board certification in basic speciality to be eligible to obtain the Subspecialty Certificate in Surgery.[15]

Finally, becoming a member of the prestigious ASSH has its own unique set of challenges. To become an active member, the candidate must have passed the Subspeciality certificate. Although the Subspeciality certificate is not needed to become an "International member," the candidate must reside outside the United States.[16] Unfortunately, the specialist IMGs practicing in the United States do not fit in either of these categories. These IMGs, even if they are board-certified via the academic route, are ineligible for ASSH membership. However, in special circumstances, exemption from the Subspeciality certificate can be obtained if two-thirds of the members of the Council determine that the individual has made extraordinary contributions to the understanding and treatment of disorders of the upper limb and/or the education and training of physicians in Hand Surgery.[16] The American Association for Hand Surgery (AAHS), while requiring board certification, does not require the Subspeciality certificate for its membership.[17]

Another overlooked aspect in an IMG's journey is family. Some IMGs enter the United States leaving behind loved ones, whereas some bring their dependents with them. Both scenarios have their own challenges. Maintaining long-distance relationships during hectic residency or fellowship training is difficult for anyone and even more so when loved ones live across the globe in a different time zone. A trip home can be expensive, and time-consuming, and returning to the United States often requires a new visa. To avoid these hassles, IMGs do not visit their home for many years. The spouses of IMG physicians are considered dependents and need special employment authorizations to work, or to obtain training. Cultural and language barriers can be challenging for children to assimilate into schools. Thus, it can be truly said that the success of an IMG stands atop the sacrifices made by the whole family.

Despite the multitude of challenges, IMGs continue to contribute to the healthcare system in the United States and to the field of Hand Surgery. From filling the gap of health-care shortage, to serving in underserved areas, and bringing in expertise, skill sets, leadership, and innovation. It will be prudent to say that Hand Surgery in the United States has greatly benefitted from the contributions of IMGs.

DISCLOSURE

No disclosures.

REFERENCES

1. Residency Application Requirements for International Medical Graduates. Aafp.org. https://www.aafp.org/students-residents/medical-students/become-a-resident/applying-to-residency/international-medical-graduates.html. [Accessed 20 May 2022].
2. Kowarski I. What to Know About International Medical Schools. 2020. Available at: https://www.usnews.com/; https://www.usnews.com/education/best-graduate-schools/top-medical-schools/articles/what-to-know-about-caribbean-medical-schools.
3. National Resident Matching Program. Advance data tables: 2022 Main Residency Match. https://www.nrmp.org/wp-content/uploads/2022/03/Advance-Data-Tables-2022-FINAL.pdf. [Accessed 20 May 2022].
4. Match Results Statistics. Nrmp.org. 2021. https://www.nrmp.org/wp-content/uploads/2021/11/Hand-Surgery_AY22.pdf.pdf. [Accessed 20 May 2022].
5. Accreditation Council for Graduate Medical Education. ACGME Common Program Requirements (Residency). https://www.acgme.org/globalassets/PFAssets/ProgramRequirements/263_363_443_HandSurgery_2020.pdf. [Accessed 27 May 2022].
6. Applying for a CMKI Fellowship | Christine M. Kleinert Institute for Hand and Micro Surgery. https://christinemkleinertinstitute.org/fellowships/applying-for-a-cmki-fellowship/. [Accessed 1 June 2022].
7. Ganga Medical Centre & Hospitals Pvt Ltd. Gangahospital.com. https://www.gangahospital.com/plastic_fellowships. [Accessed 1 June 2022].
8. Jones NF. 2016 ASSH Presidential Address: Teaching Hands-Pass It On. J Hand Surg Am 2018;43(7):591–605.
9. Waiver of the Exchange Visitor Two-Year Home-Country Physical Presence Requirement. Travel.state.gov. https://travel.state.gov/content/travel/en/us-visas/study/exchange/waiver-of-the-exchange-visitor.html. [Accessed 5 June 2022].
10. Bier D. 1.4 Million Skilled Immigrants in Employment-Based Green Card Backlogs in 2021 Cato.org. 2022. https://www.cato.org/blog/14-million-skilled-immigrants-employment-based-green-card-backlogs-2021. [Accessed 5 June 2022].
11. Policy For Exceptional Surgeons With International Training. The American Board of Plastic Surgery, Inc.. 2015. https://www.abplasticsurgery.org/media/9370/Exceptional-Surgeons-with-International-Training-approved-updated-11-2015-L.pdf. [Accessed 10 June 2022].
12. Rules And Procedures For Residency Education, Part I, And Part II Examinations. American Board of Orthopaedic Surgery. 2022. https://www.abos.org/wp-content/uploads/2022/05/Part-I-and-II-RP-2022_05_11.pdf. [Accessed 10 June 2022].
13. Academic Pathway to ABS Certification for International Medical Graduates | American Board of Surgery. https://www.absurgery.org/default.jsp?academicpathway. [Accessed 10 June 2022].
14. FSMB | State Specific Requirements for Initial Medical Licensure. Fsmb.org. 2022. https://www.fsmb.org/step-3/state-licensure/. [Accessed 10 June 2022].
15. Subspecialty Certificate in Hand Surgery of the Hand. Assh.org. 2022. https://www.assh.org/s/subspecialty-certificate-hand-surgery. [Accessed 10 June 2022].
16. Become a Member. Assh.org. 2022. https://www.assh.org/s/become-a-member. [Accessed 10 June 2022].
17. AAHS - Active Membership. American Association for Hand Surgery. https://handsurgery.org/join/active.cgi. [Accessed 15 June 2022].

Microaggressions and Implicit Bias in Hand Surgery

Kashyap Komarraju Tadisina, MD, Kelly Bettina Currie, MD*

KEYWORDS

• Implicit bias • Microaggression • Intersectionality • Hand surgery • Academic surgery • Surgery

KEY POINTS

- *Implicit bias* is an unconscious, automatic association that is either disadvantageous or favorable toward a person or group.
- A *microaggression* is an intentional or unintentional statement or action that is perceived as discriminatory against a marginalized community, emanating as the product of bias.
- *Intersectionality* is a concept that describes the exponential discrimination toward individuals who belong to more than one marginalized group, such as their racial and ethnic group and gender affiliation.
- Implicit bias and microaggressions that negatively affect marginalized groups are ubiquitous in medicine (including Hand Surgery), which contribute to health and health care disparities for patients, as well as poor representation and burnout of marginalized groups within the medical community.
- Although awareness is the first step to combating bias and microaggressions, active steps should be taken to minimize the negative effects of these phenomenon, starting with taking an implicit bias test to understand your own biases.

INTRODUCTION

Implicit bias and microaggressions are well-established principles in psychology supported by increasing amounts of empirical evidence.[1,2] Researchers have investigated several different environments to reveal how implicit bias affects large-scale organizations, business ventures, and interpersonal relationships across a variety of settings.[3,4]

Research on health care disparities has grown significantly in recent years, revealing consistent themes of inequalities in access to care and clinical outcomes associated with racial and ethnic minority groups, individuals of lower socioeconomic status, and residents of defined geographic areas.[5,6] Within medicine, findings of disparities related to race, gender, and sexual orientation have also been found in the training environment. One of the main factors contributing to these findings is underlying bias.[7] Societal standards have transformed biases in our daily lives to be less explicit, manifesting instead as implicit bias and microaggressions and other more subtle forms of discrimination and bias.[8] Implicit bias has been shown to affect patient care decision making in physicians with correlation of levels of bias and lower quality of care.[9]

Hand Surgery, with an eclectic patient mix and a group of providers who are often working in multidisciplinary teams, also has evidence of disparities in patient care and education that is founded in bias. Academic societies are in the process of focusing on addressing these issues for practicing surgeons and trainees.[10]

Department of Surgery, Division of Plastic and Reconstructive Surgery, Washington University in St. Louis School of Medicine, 660 South Euclid Avenue, St Louis, MO 63110, USA
* Corresponding author.
E-mail address: kcurrie@wustl.edu

Hand Clin 39 (2023) 95–102
https://doi.org/10.1016/j.hcl.2022.08.007

The authors aim to provide definitions and enhance awareness of implicit bias and microaggressions, highlight areas in Hand Surgery that manifest these issues, summarize relevant literature, and provide a practical evidence-based framework to guide surgeons in their practices.

DEFINITIONS AND BACKGROUND

Implicit bias is an unconscious, automatic association that is either disadvantageous or favorable toward a person or group. Although prejudice is not a new concept, implicit bias defines biases that are uncontrollable, intuitive, and irrational. Implicit bias can present itself as a preference, leading to outcomes that undermine trust. Although societal standards have evolved to disfavor explicit bias, implicit bias is harder to recognize even by the recipient.[8] There is evidence that implicit bias favoring in-groups and dominant groups and also disfavoring out-groups develops as early as 6 years old.[11,12]

A *microaggression* is a statement or action, conscious or unconscious, that is perceived as discriminatory against a marginalized community, the product of implicit bias. Originally defined in 1970 by Dr Chester Pierce to describe subtle forms of racism in the post-Jim Crow era,[13] it has evolved as discrimination has become more subtle, and it spans across multiple target groups, whether based on race, gender, sexuality, or other marginalized groups.[8] Microaggressions are admittedly difficult to navigate because they can be subjective in nature and interpretation. There are 4 defined forms of microaggression that are summarized in the following discussion, and in **Table 1** where examples are provided[14,15]:

1. Microassault: Discriminatory action or comment that is intentionally performed/spoken; however, it may not be meant to be offensive.
2. Microinsult: Unconscious verbal or nonverbal subtle rudeness or insensitivity that demeans a person's identity.
3. Microinvalidations: Unconscious acts or words that negate, undermine, or nullify the feelings and reality of a marginalized person/group.
4. Environmental microaggressions: Systemic rules or physical environments that exclude, underpin vulnerability, and perpetuate inequity.

Implicit bias and microaggression by themselves or in combination affect the individuals involved and the relationship between them. Regardless of who is affected, in the context of Hand Surgery, patient care can be compromised.

The term *intersectionality* was first coined in 1989 by Kimberlé Crenshaw, a Professor of Law at Columbia University, and a distinguished Professor of Law at the University of California, Los Angeles.[16] Intersectionality is a concept that describes the exponential discrimination toward individuals who belong to more than 1 marginalized group, such as their racial and ethnic group and gender affiliation. These individuals are often the subjects of prejudice on a larger scale due to the existence of their multiple realities. For example, a black woman who is discriminated against for being black and for being a woman will suffer more discrimination and inequity than a Black man or White woman.[17]

DISCUSSION

Hand surgeons experience multiple types of interpersonal encounters across a variety of environments. These encounters include varying levels of power and authority and situations that capture biases and microaggressions. The patient-surgeon, surgeon-peer, surgeon-staff, and surgery training environment all afford their own unique sets of challenges when it comes to addressing biases in the workplace (**Table 2**).

Patient-Surgeon Relationship

Within the Hand Surgery clinical sphere, the patient-surgeon relationship is essential in diagnosis, surgical decision-making, overall care delivery, and complication prevention and mitigation. Multiple treatment options can be available based on the condition being treated. The development of trust between the patient and surgeon is crucial in finding the care plan best suited for the patient.

Socioeconomic status has been found to affect access to hand specialty care in the United States,[18] with less access to hand trauma and congenital hand care in underserved areas.[19,20] Large-scale studies of implicit bias in health care have found evidence of health care providers displaying bias that favors patients of upper socioeconomic status,[21] by surgeons and nurses[22,23]; this cultivates a system whereby hand surgeons at tertiary referral centers facilitate care for this population.

Race-related disparities in health care are also documented in patient counseling,[24] timing of operations,[25] and perception of pain and prescription of opioids.[26,27] Unsurprisingly, patients are more likely to choose racial- and ethnic-concordant physicians[28] and are also more likely to follow their physician's recommendations if they are of the same race and ethnicity.[29]

Table 1
Types of microaggressions

Type	Definition	Examples
Microassaults	Discriminatory action or comment that is intentionally performed/ spoken; however, it may or may not have been meant to be offensive	• Using racial epithets • Telling homophobic jokes • Crossing the street and clutching their purse in the presence of individuals of low socioeconomic status
Microinsults	Unconscious verbal or nonverbal communications that convey subtle rudeness or insensitivity that demeans a person's identity	• Assuming a female is in a more junior role • Touching someone's hair without permission • Commenting on how articulate someone is given their race
Microinvalidations	Unconscious acts or words that negate, undermine, or nullify the feelings and reality of a marginalized person/group	• Mistaking a person for someone else of the same race • Stating a hurtful comment was not meant to be hurtful • Giving credit for work done by an individual with a disability to someone without a disability
Environmental Microaggressions	Systemic rules or physical environment that excludes, underpins vulnerability, and perpetuates inequity	• Lack of representation on governing bodies • Surgeons' lounge connected to male locker room, and staff lounge connected to female locker room • Naming buildings on a college campus after only White heterosexual upper class males

Implicit bias and microaggressions are multidirectional and often occur from the patient to the physician. These "contra-power" microaggressions can lead to burnout among physicians.[30] In addition, these biases are reflected in patient satisfaction scores. Metrics like these, such as Press-Ganey scores, often influence physician compensation and promotion, worsening the impact of disparities in academic medicine.[31]

Surgeon and Peers

Within the surgical community, implicit gender bias is well documented. Large cohort implicit association test (IAT) has found that among surgeons, men are associated with surgery and women with family medicine as specialties. Furthermore, cumulative implicit bias can have an impact on personnel hiring decision making. Downstream effects of such decisions are thought to contribute to underrepresentation and disparities in access to mentorship and leadership opportunities. Within Hand Surgery, documented downstream disparities in research,[32,33] society leadership,[34] and hand fellowship directorship[35] have been noted.

Surgeon and Staff

As a surgeon in the health care environment, one interacts with many types of staff as an integral part of the operating room team. A recent validated survey study found that surgeons' leadership behaviors affected intraoperative team performance, particularly negative behaviors.[36] Both in and out of the operating room, hand surgeons encounter administrative, nursing, technical, cleaning, and supply chain team members on a daily basis. Members of each of these groups have their own separate dynamics and propensity for biases.

Studies on operating room staff characteristics that were predictive of surgeons being written up have found that the likelihood of writing up the surgeon was predicted by role, with technologists, nurses, and assistants reporting surgeons at higher frequencies.[37]

Furthermore, the age/generation of operating room staff and how they interpreted surgeons'

Table 2
Summary of bias and clinical microaggression for the hand surgeon

Environments	Examples of Implicit Biases	Examples of Clinical Microaggression
Surgeon-patient	Disfavor for patients who make below the federal poverty line Preference for males	• Patients with incomes below federal poverty level being denied care because the provider knows they cannot pay • Patients being late due to taking multiple public transportations are labeled as "rude" for being late to appointments • Patient calling the male medical student "Doctor" and the female attending "Honey"
Surgeon-peer	Disfavor for Black community Preference for neurotypical	• A surgeon telling a peer "One of my good friends is black," to prove they are not biased • A surgeon with ADHD is ridiculed for never listening at faculty meetings
Surgeon-staff	Preference for White Preference for males Disfavor of homosexuality	• The OR nurse mistakes the new black female attending as a medical student • A male floor nurse says "no homo" after a gay surgeon compliments his haircut
Training environment	Disfavor for heterosexuality Preference for males Disfavor for Latino/a community	• A program director asks a homosexual male resident what his "wife thinks" of him working long hours • Latina medical student is asked "Are you sure you want to go into surgery?"

Abbreviations: ADHD, attention-deficit hyperactivity disorder; OR, operating room.

behavior has revealed that older generations were more likely to find behaviors of impatience, tardiness, and swearing to be inappropriate compared with younger generations who found fault with deviation from rules and regulations such as the surgical time out.[38]

The microaggression of mislabeling a physician from a marginalized group as someone who has less training (mistaking a female attending for a nurse, or a black resident as the janitorial staff) occurs frequently. However, the physician is faced with a dilemma because speaking up about the microaggression may be perceived as disrespect for the nonphysician staff and their profession.[30]

At the crux of these observations is the lack of insight into one's own biases. For instance, survey studies of nurses at an academic hospital found that whereas 71% of those surveyed believed they had no implicit bias, in actuality, only 14% displayed no implicit bias after taking an IAT regarding clinical vignette scenarios.[23]

Often, being the leader of their team during these times, hand surgeons must be aware of role-specific, generational, race, ethnicity, and socioeconomic biases and microaggressions.

Training Environment

The academic training environment has lent itself to several studies regarding the presence of both bias and microaggressions, providing insight into training programs within medical settings. Although most studies have unanimous themes, the frequency and consistency may provide evidence that biases are being encouraged and facilitated within our training programs.

Several recent reports have found disparities and bias manifesting in Hand Surgery letters of recommendations[39] and Orthopedic Surgery residency interviews.[40] A recent survey study of Plastic Surgery trainees found that 69% of trainees reported experiencing microaggressions within the past year, with females, racial, and sexual minorities having higher odds of reporting such experiences.[41]

Furthermore, there is some consensus that as a trainee, the risk of reporting racial discrimination is not worth the reward of potential equity.[42] Hence, as leaders of a training program, surgical team, operating room, or administrative teams, one must be increasingly aware of how their actions may be interpreted.

Intersectionality has been shown to be relevant in the graduation rates of General Surgery residents. A study by Keshinro and colleagues[17] demonstrated that the increase in women graduates of General Surgery residencies is attributed in most part to the increase in White and Asian women, and not black and Latina women; this occurs despite an increasing number of black and Latina women applicants to General Surgery residency.[17]

Attrition of trainees from surgical training is more common in women and racial/ethnic minorities.[17,43,44] This attrition has been reported to be associated with burnout that is secondary to implicit bias and microaggressions.[45,46] The attrition of trainees with minority backgrounds perpetuates the deficiency of diversity among the ranks of practicing surgeons and is detrimental to patient care.

Action Plan

At an institutional level, many organizations are incorporating Diversity, Equity, and Inclusion committees or including curricula within medical education to prepare health care providers to be more aware and trained regarding implicit biases.[47] These organizations can be great resources to find and take an IAT, provide training for one's teams, and gain exposure through events and lectures. However, ultimate change must come at the individual level, and these are the efforts on which the authors focus, with strategies summarized in **Table 3**.

For those striving to work through strategies to reduce implicit biases and microagressions in the workplace, definitions and evidence of existing problems only help to some extent. Although there is no true way to eliminate implicit bias from our decision making, minimizing its negative impact on others is an achievable goal. Although awareness is the first step to solution, implementing change to reduce bias is often harder than it seems.

In psychology literature, it is well known that small changes in behavior can cumulatively bring about change. For example, it is encouraging to note research establishing that implicit bias is a habit that can be broken. Devine and colleagues[48]

Table 3
Strategies to combat implicit bias and microaggressions

Strategy Source	Explanation	Useful Link
Project Implicit[49]	Take an IAT	https://www.projectimplicit.net
APA's recommendations for the target, bystander, or microaggressor[50]	Target: • Consider the context • Take care of yourself • Don't be fooled by microaggressions packaged as opportunities ("Minority tax") Bystander: • Be an ally • Speak for yourself Microaggressor: • Try not to be defensive • Acknowledge the other person is hurt • Apologize and reflect	https://www.apa.org/monitor/2017/01/microaggressions
APA's Inclusive Language Guidelines[51]	Consciously avoid using language that may be perceived as a microaggression, regardless of the intent	https://www.apa.org/about/apa/equity-diversity-inclusion/language-guidelines

Abbreviation: APA, American Psychological Association.

developed an intervention to reduce implicit bias and showed that it is possible to retain this gain over a 12-week period. The American Psychology Association has a concise outlined plan for the parties involved in any microaggression and is summarized in **Table 3**. The following section lists the action steps or behaviors that health care providers can practice to reduce the potential for displaying implicit bias and microaggressions.

CLINICS CARE POINTS

- Educate yourself and be aware of how your interactions are perceived by those you interact with as a surgeon (see **Tables 1** and **2**).
- Take an implicit bias test and be receptive to the results of the test[22] and critically think about your background and your own potential preferences (see **Table 3**).
- Ask patients "What's going on in your world right now and how is your hand problem affecting it?" instead of "How's your hand doing"?
- At the end of any encounter, ask patients if they feel comfortable instead of asking if they understand what you are saying.
- Offer a second opinion and be open to patients not wanting to seek care with you. Everybody is not for everybody.
- Facilitate a training session for team members and trainees.
  - Provide scenarios that do and do not depict implicit bias and ask respondents to react and differentiate between the 2 scenarios.
  - Provide scenarios of different types of implicit bias/microaggression and ask the respondent to select from options about how the target should respond.
  - Vary the scenarios so that the recipient of the bias/microaggression has more power or less power (eg, staff member on surgeon).
- Listen to others and explore why something was perceived as hurtful or demeaning, even if that was not the intention.
- Strive to use inclusive language to avoid conscious and unconscious microaggressions (see **Table 3**),

SUMMARY

The existence and detriment of implicit bias and microaggressions is becoming more and more recognized in medicine. Awareness of these psychological attacks is not enough to mitigate or stop them from occurring, or prevent the progression of their downstream effects. As hand surgeons, we can be leaders in our medical community and actively work to eliminate these learned but entrenched views of others. Resources are available to guide and support us through this process and spearhead a culture change within our subspecialized field of medicine.

REFERENCES

1. Greenwald AG, McGhee DE, Schwartz JKL. Measuring individual differences in implicit cognition: The implicit association test. J Pers Soc Psychol 1998;74:1464–80.
2. Sue DW. Microaggressions in everyday life: race, gender, and sexual orientation. Hoboken, NJ: John Wiley & Sons, Inc.; 2010.
3. Greenwald AG, McGhee DE, Schwartz JKL. Measuring individual differences in implicit cognition: the implicit association test. J Pers Soc Psychol 2003;85(2):197–216.
4. Sue DW. Microaggressions and "evidence": empirical or experiential reality? Perspect Psychol Sci 2017;12(1):170–2.
5. Baxter NB, Howard JC, Chung KC. A systematic review of health disparities research in plastic surgery. Plast Reconstr Surg 2021;147(3):529–37.
6. Green AR, Carney DR, Pallin DJ, et al. Implicit bias among physicians and its prediction of thrombolysis decisions for black and white patients. J Gen Intern Med 2007;22(9):1231–8.
7. Saluja B, Bryant Z. How implicit bias contributes to racial disparities in maternal morbidity and mortality in the United States. J Womens Health (Larchmt) 2021;30(2):270–3.
8. Turner J, Higgins R, Childs E. Microaggression and Implicit Bias. Am Surg 2021;87(11):1727–31.
9. FitzGerald C, Hurst S. Implicit bias in healthcare professionals: a systematic review. BMC Med Ethics 2017;18(1):19.
10. Overland MK, Zumsteg JM, Lindo EG, et al. Microaggressionsin Clinical Training and Practice. PMR 2019;11(9):1004–12.
11. Dunham Y, Baron AS, Banaji MR. The development of implicit intergroup cognition. Trends Cogn Sci 2008;(12):248–53.
12. Baron AS, Banaji MR. The development of implicit attitudes. Evidence of race evaluations from ages 6 and 10 and adulthood. Psychol Sci 2006;17(1):53–8.
13. Pierce CM. Black psychiatry one year after Miami. J Natl Med Assoc 1970;62(6):471–3.
14. Sue DW, Capodilupo CM, Torino GC, et al. Racial microaggressions in everyday life: implications for clinical practice. Am Psychol 2007;62(4):271–86.

15. Torres MB, Salles A, Cochran A. Recognizing and Reacting to Microaggressions in Medicine and Surgery. JAMA Surg 2019;154(9):868–72.
16. Crenshaw K. Demarginalizing the intersection of race and sex: a black feminist critique of antidiscrimination doc-trine, feminist theory and antiracist politics. Univ Chic LegForum; 1989. p. 139–67.
17. Keshinro A, Butler P, Fayanju O, et al. Examination of intersectionality and the pipeline for black academic surgeons. JAMA Surg 2022;157(4):327–34.
18. Rios-Diaz AJ, Metcalfe D, Singh M, et al. Inequalities in Specialist Hand Surgeon Distribution across the United States. Plast Reconstr Surg 2016;137(5): 1516–22.
19. Anthony JR, Poole VN, Sexton KW, et al. Tennessee emergency hand care distributions and disparities: Emergent hand care disparities. Hand (N Y). 2013; 8(2):172–8.
20. Kalmar CL, Drolet BC. Socioeconomic Disparities in Surgical Care for Congenital Hand Differences. Hand (N Y) 2022. https://doi.org/10.1177/15589447221092059. 15589447221092059.
21. Salles A, Awad M, Goldin L, et al. Estimating implicit and explicit gender bias among health care professionals and surgeons. JAMA Netw Open 2019;2(7): e196545.
22. Dossa F, Baxter NN. Implicit Bias in Surgery-Hiding in Plain Sight. JAMA Netw Open 2019;2(7):e196535.
23. Haider AH, Schneider EB, Sriram N, et al. Unconscious race and class biases among registered nurses: vignette-based study using implicit association testing. J Am Coll Surg 2015;220(6):1077–86.e3.
24. Menendez ME, van Hoorn BT, Mackert M, et al. Patients with limited health literacy ask fewer questions during office visits with hand surgeons. Clin Orthop Relat Res 2017;475:1291–7.
25. Bucknor A, Huang A, Wu W, et al. Socioeconomic disparities inbrachial plexus surgery: a national database analysis. Plast Reconstr Surg Glob Open 2019;7:E2118.
26. Hoffman KM, Trawalter S, Axt JR, et al. Racial bias in pain assessment and treatment recommendations, and false beliefs about biological differences between blacks and whites. Proc Natl Acad Sci U S A 2016;113:4296–301.
27. Bradford PS, Dacus AR, Chhabra AB, et al. How to Be An Antiracist Hand Surgery Educator. J Hand Surg Am 2021;46(6):507–11.
28. Saha S, Taggart SH, Komaromy M, et al. Do patients choose physicians of their own race? Health Aff (Millwood) 2000;19(4):76–83.
29. Murray-García JL, García JA, Schembri ME, et al. The service patterns of a racially, ethnically, and linguistically diverse housestaff. Acad Med 2001; 76(12):1232–2124.
30. Ahmad SR, Ahmad TR, Balasubramanian V, et al. Are you really the doctor? Physician Experiences with Gendered Microaggressions from Patients. J Womens Health (Larchmt) 2022;31(4):521–32.
31. Rogo-Gupta LJ, Haunschild C, Altamirano J, et al. Physician gender is associated with press ganey patient satisfaction scores in outpatient gynecology. Womens Health Issues 2018;28(3):281–5.
32. Kalliainen LK, Wisecarverl, Cummings A, et al. Sex bias in hand surgery research. J Hand Surg Am 2018;43(11):1026–9.
33. Xu RF, Varady NH, Chen AF, et al. Gender disparity trends in authorship of hand surgery research. J Hand Surg Am 2022;47(5):420–8.
34. Brisbin AK, Chen W, Goldschmidt E, et al. Gender diversity in hand surgery leadership. Hand (N Y). 2022. 15589447211038679.
35. Schiller NC, Spielman AF, Sama AJ, et al. Leadership trends at hand surgery fellowships. Hand (N Y). 2022. https://doi.org/10.1177/15589447211073977. 15589447211073977.
36. Barling J, Akers A, Beiko D. The impact of positive and negative intraoperative surgeons' leadership behaviors on surgical team performance. Am J Surg 2018;215(1):14–8.
37. Corsini EM, Luc JGY, Mitchell KG, et al. Predictors of the response of operating room personnel to surgeon behaviors. Surg Today 2019;49(11): 927–35.
38. Luc JGY, Corsini EM, Mitchell KG, et al. Effect of operating room personnel generation on perceptions and responses to surgeon behavior. Am Surg 2021;87(12):1934–45.
39. Bradford PS, Akyeampong D, Fleming MA 2nd, et al. Racial and gender discrimination in hand surgery letters of recommendation. J Hand Surg Am 2021; 46(11):998–1005.e2.
40. Webber CRJ, Davie R, Herzwurm Z, et al. Is There unconscious bias in the orthopaedic residency interview selection process? J Surg Educ 2022. S1931-7204(22)00017-4.
41. Goulart MF, Huayllani MT, Balch Samora J, et al. Assessing the prevalence of microaggressions in plastic surgery training: a national survey. Plast Reconstr Surg Glob Open 2021;9(12):e4062.
42. Fleming MA 2nd, Scott EJ, Bradford PS, et al. The risk and reward of speaking out for racial equity in surgical training. J Surg Educ 2021;78(5): 1387–92.
43. Bauer JM, Holt GE. National orthopedic residency attrition: who is at risk? J Surg Educ 2016;73(5): 852–7.
44. Yeo HL, Abelson JS, Symer MM, et al. Association of time to attrition in surgical residency with individual resident and programmatic factors. JAMA Surg 2018;153(6):511–7.
45. Aryee JNA, Bolarinwa SA, Montgomery SR Jr, et al. Race, gender, and residency: a survey of trainee experience. J Natl Med Assoc 2021;113(2):199–207.

46. Sudol NT, Guaderrama NM, Honsberger P, et al. Prevalence and nature of sexist and racial/ethnic microaggressions against surgeons and anesthesiologists. JAMA Surg 2021;156(5):e210265.
47. Sukhera J, Watling C. A framework for integrating implicit bias recognition into health professions education. Acad Med 2018;93(1):35–40.
48. Devine PG, Forscher PS, Austin AJ, et al. Long-term reduction in implicit race bias: a prejudice habit-breaking intervention. J Exp Soc Psychol 2012;48: 1267–78.
49. Project implicit. Available at. https://www.projectimplicit.net/. Accessed June 15, 2022.
50. Clay RA. Did you really just say that?. In: Monitor psychol, 48 2017. Available at: https://www.apa.org/monitor/2017/01/microaggressions; 2017. Accessed June 15, 2022.
51. American Psychological Association. Inclusive language guidelines. 2021. Available at: https://www.apa.org/about/apa/equity-diversity-inclusion/language-guidelines. Accessed: June 15, 2022.

Allyship for Diversity, Equity, and Inclusion in Hand Surgery

Shea Ray, MD, MS, Jennifer D'Auria, MD, Hannah Lee, MD, Mark Baratz, MD*

KEYWORDS

- Allyship • Diversity • Inclusion

KEY POINTS

- Diversity among hand surgeons can be realized with active support by allies in positions of influence.
- Great allies listen, learn, and act.
- The skills required to enhance your capabilities as an ally are accessible through a number of our professional organizations.

DEFINITION OF ALLYSHIP

Merriam Webster defines allyship as the state or condition of being an ally. Leaving the definition at this may imply that it is only a label. Delving deeper, "ally" is a noun and verb. In its most simplistic terms, allyship is a helper supporting another entity. In the context of diversity initiatives, allyship has been more clearly defined as "an active, consistent, and arduous practice of unlearning and re-evaluating, in which a person in a position of privilege and power seeks to operate in solidarity with a marginalized group."[1] This definition requires that allies must recognize that they are in a majority status and that affords them the power to support, promote, and help those in the nonmajority; this entails an educated assessment of the environment in which one interacts with others and knowledge about the challenges that marginalized groups can encounter. Perhaps more importantly, beyond identification as an ally, the ally must intentionally act in support of the nonmajority, and this demands open dialogue between the marginalized and nonmarginalized in what to do and how to do it.

HISTORY OF ALLYSHIP

The first published use of the word allyship dates to 1849; however, it was not used in the modern sense of the word. In 1943 Albert Hamilton wrote about how allies may help with the fight for racial equality.[2] Since the 1970s, supporters of the LGBTQIA+ (Lesbian, Gay, Bisexual, Transgender, Queer or Questioning, Intersex, Asexual, and More) community have been identified as allies. As discussed earlier, allyship is not just labeling oneself as an ally. The more modern definition of identification, solidarity, action, promotion, and adjustment is more a recent construct. In fact, allyship was added to dictionary.com in 2021. That same year, it was also given the recognition of Word of the Year.[3]

In business, many companies have a dedicated division that focuses on initiatives of diversity, equity, and inclusion. All the top 5 Fortune 500

Department of Orthopaedics, University of Pittsburgh Medical Center, 2000 Oxford Drive – Suite 510, Bethel Park, PA 15102, USA
* Corresponding author.
E-mail address: baratzme@upmc.edu

Hand Clin 39 (2023) 103–109
https://doi.org/10.1016/j.hcl.2022.08.008

companies: Walmart, Amazon, Apple, CVS Health, and UnitedHealth Group have these divisions.[4] It is less clear on how allyship is incorporated because this term is not on the front-facing resource pages for these divisions. This situation may change as the concept of allyship takes a more prominent role in social justice. For example, Google has an allyship program that aims to provide employees with knowledge, resources, and ways to enact allyship in their profession.[5]

Within health care, there is similar room for growth in discussing, learning about, and incorporating allyship. At the time of writing, there are no currently published articles discussing allyship in the *Journal of Hand Surgery*, the official journal of the American Society for Surgery of the Hand. In the *Journal of the American Academy of Orthopedic Surgeons*, there is 1 article on the topic. In the *New England Journal of Medicine*, there are 4 articles mentioning allyship.

EVIDENCE FOR WHY ALLYSHIP IS HELPFUL AND NEEDED

In business, putting the intangible benefits aside, diversity can increase financial productivity. The success rate of acquisitions and initial public offerings of partners with shared ethnicity was 26.4% compared with that of nonhomogeneous partnerships at 32.2%. Venture capital firms have notoriously low rates of diversity. When venture capital firms increased the percentage of female partners by 10%, fund returns grew by 1.5%.[6]

In health care, it is important that physicians reflect the diverse population for whom they are caring for. In Orthopedic Surgery, there has been a consistent lack of diversity of gender, race, and sexual orientation. Nth Dimensions is a nonprofit organization that seeks to provide exposure, opportunity, and mentorship to underrepresented students in medicine. Part of their process to ensure diversity and equity includes training in allyship. The outcomes of participating in Nth Dimensions are impressive. Women and unrepresented minorities are, respectively, 45 and 15 times more likely to apply to Orthopedic Surgery residency.[7] In addition, the match rate is 92% for those in the program compared with the national average of 77%.[7] There are data to show that even modest programs can effect change. Workshops less than 2 hours on allyship for graduate medical trainees have been shown to significantly increase knowledge and comprehension of allyship.[7]

What Makes a Good Ally?

Warren and Warren[8] surveyed 14 experts identified as established leaders in their respective fields. The experts were selected from diverse backgrounds to refine the definition of and criteria for an exemplary ally.[8] Their definition and criteria for exemplary allies are those who:

1. Tap into their values to support optimal functioning of marginalized group members
2. Listen to, give credence to, and amplify the voices of marginalized group members
3. Offer support in ways marginalized group members share is in their best interest
4. Are committed to staying informed about critical experiences of marginalized groups
5. Make space for marginalized groups in places they are not yet occupying
6. Go beyond sympathy and "get in the trenches" to work with marginalized groups
7. Have a disposition to act according to their ideals of allyship across life domains
8. Affirm their acts and express the principles and the moral rationale underlying the acts
9. Possess a willingness to risk their self-interest for the sake of their values of allyship
10. Leverage their privilege to inspire other privileged group members to allyship action

Similarly, Bourke and Espedido[9] surveyed more than 4100 employees about inclusion. The 6 traits that distinguished inclusive leaders included the following:

1. Visible commitment: Articulates authentic commitment to diversity, challenges status quo, and accepts accountability
2. Humility: Admits mistakes and creates space for others to contribute
3. Awareness of bias: Works to build awareness of personal blind spots and to ensure meritocracy
4. Curiosity about others: Demonstrates an open mindset with deep curiosity. Listens without judgment
5. Cultural intelligence: Attentive to others' cultures and adapts as required
6. Effective collaboration: Empowers others and provides psychological safety

How do You Become a Good Ally?

There is no single, agreed-upon set of behaviors. Salter and Migliaccio[10] proposed allyship behaviors and processes as 3 broad categories: knowledge and awareness, communication and confrontation, and action and advocacy.

Knowledge and awareness

Allies must be aware of and educate themselves about the experiences of marginalized group members. In the context of gender, male allies must learn to recognize sexism when it occurs. For the LGBTQIA+ community, it can entail learning to separate myth from fact. Understanding minority experiences needs to include the role the majority population plays in the minority experiences—intentional or unintentional. White people need to understand institutional racism, White privilege, and their own biases to truly be allies to people of different race.

Communication and confrontation

Although knowledge and awareness are important, an ally should communicate with others about these issues. The ally must actively participate and initiate in discussions about ways to promote minority rights. These communications should be public for others to witness. Confrontation is one means to challenge prejudice and discrimination in others; it can lead to positive change and breaks down the "bystander effect."

Action and advocacy

Allies support and promote minority communities. Allies can provide tangible benefits to minority populations. Allies can help introduce minority-supportive ideas into their organizations, particularly within the leadership circle. Allies can educate people on minority issues and persuade others to change their minds. Allies can support minorities directly. Sometimes a simple act of kindness is invaluable.

Melaku and colleagues,[18] described evidence-based best practices for becoming an ally in their recent Harvard Business Review article "Be a Better Ally." Although their advice was addressed largely to White men, it applies to anyone in a privileged group who is striving for an inclusive organization. Their proposed steps are as follows:

1. *Educate yourself:* It can be emotionally and cognitively exhausting for marginalized group members to bear the load of teaching you about their experiences with inequality and injustice. A good ally takes the initiative to read, listen, watch, and deepen their understanding. Request permission when asking others about their experiences. Recognize that the members of a marginalized group may not all have the same experiences; this is especially true if they are of different marginalized cohorts. A good example is that White women's experiences are not necessarily similar to those of women of color. Generalization from 1 or 2 colleagues' experience should be avoided. In addition, do not rely too heavily on your own experience. The perspective of a White male surgeon will not mirror that of a marginalized female surgeon. Finally, transform your perspective as a leader by staying alert to inequities and disparities. Pay attention to marginalized group members' experience in meetings and gatherings—"Once you put on that lens, you can't take it off. The world never looks the same."[18]
2. *Own your privilege:* Being an ally requires recognizing the privileges that others have been overtly or subtly denied. Although it can be painful to admit that you have not entirely earned your success, it is necessary. A White male surgeon may have never thought about how his career decision affects his wife and kids, or why he is more focusing on his career instead of his family; however, it is a frequent question for women surgeons. White men are far less likely to need to adjust their style of speech, appearance, and behavior to succeed in their workplace. This "code-switching" is extra work that takes an emotional toll for marginalized group members.
3. *Accept feedback:* Intentionally seek feedback while recognizing the power dynamics at play. The request for feedback may add invisible labor and stress to the marginalized individual when they are not in secure positions. It is important to establish trusting relationships with members from marginalized groups who will give honest feedback about your workplace conduct. Value these comments.
4. *Become a confidant:* Marginalized group members who have succeeded typically had trusting relationships with White, male leadership who took a genuine interest in their careers. Make yourself available, listen generously, and empathize and validate their experiences.
5. *Bring diversity to the table:* Marginalized group members are often the "only" ones in the room who can experience outsider and impostor feelings. These feelings can be combated by inviting more from marginalized groups to gatherings. As an ally, ask specific questions of people whose contributions and expertise are often overlooked or devalued.
6. *See something, say something:* Rather than waiting for marginalized individuals to react and then get accused of "playing the race or gender card," monitor your workplace and be decisive in shutting down racist or sexist comments and behaviors. Give your support in the moment, versus approaching the victim later to offer sympathy when you witness discrimination. Look out for gaslighting, which is a tactic used to invalidate someone's experience. Physicians have a history of gaslighting both patients and colleagues. Consider a

Nepalese woman who presents with complaints of chronic wrist pain. With a cursory examination, no radiographs, and no further workup she is dismissed as having "arthritis." She is offered over-the-counter nonsteroidal anti-inflammatory medications and no follow-up. A White man with the identical condition is diagnosed after appropriate workup with early rheumatoid arthritis. In a different scenario, think about a young female attending who musters the courage to approach her Chairman about a recurrent pattern of inappropriate comments and behavior on the part of one of her male colleagues. Without exploring the circumstance, the young attending is dismissed with "Maybe you're being oversensitive. Try being more of a team player." If you are aware of these instances, intervene whether or not the members of the marginalized group are in the room—explain that you are offended and that such comments or behaviors are not acceptable or representative of your organization. These confrontations can be framed as a learning or growth opportunity for the offender and the team. Finally, avoid the common mistake of thinking that you are absolved of your own biases and prejudices, or be an ally to put yourself on a higher moral ground.

7. *Sponsor marginalized coworkers:* Seek out talented protégés from entirely different racial and cultural background. Nominate the protégés on the basis of their potentials rather than expecting them to prove that they can do a job in advance. Introduce protégés to key players in your professional networks to open up broader set of opportunities.
8. *Insist on diverse candidates:* Pay gaps, low retention, and stalled career progression for marginalized group members are due to bias and discrimination in hiring, professional development, and promotions. For hiring, insist on open job listings and targeted recruiting versus overreliance on referrals, which leads to perpetuation of workforce homogeneity. Make sure the candidate pool is diverse. Involve members of marginalized groups in the hiring process or assign another team member to serve as a "bias interrupter."
9. *Build a community of allies:* Broaden your impact by joining or forming groups of colleagues interested in fighting racism and gender inequality.

In summary, to become a good ally, one needs to ask and listen. Listening to understand is different than listening to respond. One should join or partner with impactful groups, such as Ruth Jackson Orthopaedic Society (RJOS) and J. Robert Gladden Orthopaedic Society. One should act at home and nationally, which is particularly impactful coming from people already in leadership circle.

CONTEXTUALIZATION: PERSONAL EXAMPLES OF BENEFITTING FROM AN ALLY

Real-world and personal examples of allyship often speak louder than theorizing about how allyship should work. The following anecdotes are written by individuals who have benefitted in various ways from allies in the fields of Orthopedics and Hand Surgery.

"As a female Orthopaedic trained hand surgeon, I have found myself in the non-majority throughout my medical training in the context of my co-residents, co-fellows, attendings, and now colleagues. In reflection upon different stages of my medical career, I believe that there have been many individuals who have helped further my career, both male and female. But, there are two male attendings who played pivotal roles as an ally. When I became interested in pursuing Orthopaedic Surgery as a medical student, I felt that I did not fit the mold. Where I went to medical school, the Orthopaedic residents were mostly male, wore cowboy boots, and chewed tobacco in the call room. Fortunately, I crossed paths with an attending who was an institutional and national leader in Sports Medicine. I expressed my concerns about not fitting in, and he dispelled that worry immediately. He told me that if I chose to pursue Orthopaedic Surgery, demonstrated disciplined work ethic, and had the appropriate credentials to match to Orthopaedics, that he would support me. While his words were powerful in changing my mindset, his actions were more powerful. He acknowledged my name in research presentations and publicly recommended me for Orthopaedic Surgery residency. Moreover, he connected me to the Chair of the Department where I ultimately ended up matching for residency and am now faculty. As a resident, I again fell into a distorted mindset that Orthopaedic Surgery requires a physical strength that I was lacking as a woman. This belief led to self-doubt with respect to capability in reductions, with surgical instruments and with procedures that required force. I expressed my concern for lack of strength one day to one of the trauma surgeons. Again, he was an institutional and national leader in his field. He stopped me immediately after I said that and told me that I had strength–my strength was going to be knowledge in using instruments to my power advantage. From that day forward, I felt safe in his cases. Importantly his support was not in a vacuum. I had heard him say to other attending surgeons on multiple occasions that I had good surgical skills. His allyship re-established my confidence in the operating room; a trait that I carry to this day."

"Although I now realize how few women there are in Orthopaedics as compared to men, I have not always known those statistics. As I began choosing a career path in high school and college, I never considered myself to be someone who would benefit from allyship but have since realized that I've been the beneficiary of multiple acts of allyship (by both men and women) that have helped guide me on my path. Prior to my second round of medical school applications, the chief of vascular surgery at one of the local hospitals offered, unprompted, to help me with mock interviews. When I first started expressing interest in the field of Orthopaedics to male surgeons that I knew, it was always met with excitement and a willingness to help with shadowing experience and letters of recommendation. While in medical school, a female Orthopaedic Surgery resident sought me out in conversation at the gym; that conversation with a stranger turned into a roommate, friend, mentor, and now colleague. Finally, as a fourth-year resident attending the ASSH meeting, one of the male Hand surgeons from my institution asked me if I was going to attend the "Women in Hand Surgery" session. This surgeon attended the session with me and introduced me to the person who would become my Hand Surgery fellowship program director just a couple of years later. Each of these individuals acknowledged my goals, believed in my potential, and were willing to take the time to invest in me as a future Orthopaedic surgeon. They never emphasized the fact that I would be a minority in the field, and probably did not even think of themselves as allies in the moment. They simply saw me as someone who was committed to a goal and took action to leverage me in whatever way they knew how."

"Even as a White, male medical student I did not fit the mold. The archetype resident in my program was a collegiate wrestler or football player, preferably from an Ivy league school. A young Asian attending became my mentor, ally and accomplice. When I was accepted to the program, I heard grumblings from senior residents "why did he get in"? The Ally was Dr. Freddie Fu. I got in because he advocated vociferously on my behalf. Dr. Fu went on to create one of the more diverse Orthopedic Surgery training programs in the country. I went on to develop a sensitivity for the power of the ally."

Where Do We Go From Here?

There are numerous resources available for providers who want to take steps to exercise allyship via a formal mechanism, as well as organizations that provide opportunities for both allies and members of underrepresented groups. Although not an exhaustive list, these are well-established channels that serve as a starting point.

National level

At the national level, the American Academy of Orthopaedic Surgeons (AAOS) has included diversity as a strategic goal since 2018, with its Diversity Advisory Board in place to guide initiatives. To help track progress, the AAOS produces a Governance Diversity Report and a Diversity Dashboard Year End Review. The newly established IDEA Grant program (Inspiring Diversity, Equity, and Access) was created to provide resources for diversity, equity, and inclusion initiatives and can be applied for by any member of the Academy (www.aaos.org).

The RJOS, founded in 1983, provides a support and networking group for women orthopedic surgeons. Membership is available to women at all levels of training and practice. Men are also invited to join. RJOS hosts an annual meeting, offers a mentorship program, and has multiple committees that provide membership opportunities. Grants and scholarships for research and meeting attendance are made possible through the endowment with the Orthopaedic Research and Education Foundation (www.rjos.org).

The J. Robert Gladden Orthopaedic Society became formally incorporated as an affiliate specialty society of the AAOS in 1998 and aims to increase diversity within the orthopedic profession. Membership is open to all genders and ethnicities starting at the medical student level. Opportunities include their annual luncheon and biennial meeting, mentoring opportunities, research grants, traveling fellowships, and practice assistance (www.gladdensociety.org).

Nth Dimensions was founded in 2004 as a pipeline program to address the paucity of women and underrepresented minorities in Orthopedic Surgery. Programming includes surgeon-led lectures and workshops, medical student symposiums, and summer internships. Ninety-one percent of their scholars and affiliates have matched successfully into residency positions (www.nthdimensions.org).

Hand surgery subspecialty level

Within hand surgery, both the American Society for Surgery of the Hand (ASSH) and the American Association for Hand Surgery (AAHS) have various initiatives and programs that promote allyship. At the academic level, this includes publication of research in the *Journal of Hand Surgery* and *HAND* that touch on topics of allyship, diversity, equity, and inclusion as they relate to the field of hand surgery. At both organizations' annual meetings, instructional courses, and panels that discuss these topics have become part of regular programming. To help with these initiatives, the AAHS has a committee dedicated to Diversity, Equity, and Inclusion, and the ASSH has a Diversity Committee/Task Force. In addition, the ASSH's online platform Hand.e contains multiple lectures and seminars related to allyship, diversity, equity, and inclusion (www.assh.org, www.handsurgery.org).

Individual level

Although organizations and systems can be large contributors toward promoting allyship within Orthopedics and Hand Surgery, these larger movements are the result of individuals recognizing the importance of allyship and being committed to contributing to change. As such, the impetus to move toward allyship often comes after self-reflection, understanding biases, and being educated on topics related to allyship, DEI (Diversity, Equity, and Inclusion), and the underrepresented groups that are being advocated for. With that individual foundation in place, it then becomes easier to move toward advocating for systematic change.

At the ground level, some practical ways to pursue this individual growth are through becoming a student and testing your perceptions. What topics do you need to know more about or understand better? What are your implicit biases? How can you advocate for underrepresented groups in your daily practice? The online resource Hand.e has many lectures that can serve as launch points, including "Leadership Strategies: Women in Hand Surgery" by Dr Jennifer Wolf, "Diversity and Inclusion: How to be an Antiracist Hand Surgery Educator" with multiple authors facilitated by Dr Michael Galvez and Dr Megan Conti Mica, and "Having It All: Balancing Work and Home Demands of Being a Hand Surgeon" by Dr Julie Adams.[11–13] The Harvard Implicit Association Test can be a helpful way of identifying areas of implicit bias (www.implicit.harvard.edu), and the LGBTQ Ally Identity Measure (AIM) is a validated 19-item tool that assesses the domains of knowledge and skills, openness and support, and awareness of oppression.[14] Training that targets LGBTQ+ competency in the setting of health care has been shown to improve the AIM score among General Surgery residents and may have similar benefits when applied more broadly among other trainees and faculty.[15]

BIGGER QUESTIONS

Despite the existence of these and other supportive programs on a larger scale, there are still challenges with regard to implementation of allyship and DEI initiatives at the health system and departmental levels. Below are some questions that may be helpful to consider and discuss among colleagues and leadership before engaging in these activities:

- What do you see as the most important steps advocating for allyship, specifically in Orthopedics and Hand Surgery? At what time point are each of these steps or interventions most beneficial?
- How do you want your institution to address diversity, equity, and inclusion? Who can you talk to in your organization to make these desires known?
- The concept of a "minority tax" is well described in the literature and describes the tax of extra responsibilities placed on minority groups in the name of efforts to achieve diversity.[16] Are there undue burdens being placed on underrepresented individuals in your department/organization to carry the weight when it comes to work related to diversity?
- What is the return on this work for working toward allyship and DEI initiatives, and how can the adverse outcomes of the minority tax be reduced (i.e. removing minorities from diversity-related projects, providing protected time and/or compensation for these activities)? These are among suggested tactics proposed by Williamson and colleagues to reform the minority tax.[17]
- What steps are being taken to battle diversity leadership burnout?
- Are there adequate financial and personnel resources in place to successfully implement the desired programs and initiatives?

CLOSING THOUGHTS

Being an ally begins with belief in and passion for gardening: the process of nurturing others in groups with less representation grow to their greatest potential. It is learned and begins with the humility of one who may sense inequity but has likely not felt it. It means maintaining an attitude of continuous sensitivity to others' experience: a willingness to see the terrain through their eyes. Being open to small changes and providing opportunities is the easy part. Addressing systemic and cultural issues is more challenging and sometimes requires confrontation. Most of us hate confrontation. Confrontation may risk alienating senior physicians who are part of your support system, but do not share your vision for our Hand Surgery specialty. The costs are real, but the benefits are greater. Diversity in a garden or a medical community is the only way to ensure sustainability.

DISCLOSURE

The authors received no financial support in the creation of this article.

ACKNOWLEDGMENTS

The authors thank Dominic Coutinho for helping them put together and edit this article.

REFERENCES

1. allyship | THE ANTI-OPPRESSION NETWORK. The Anti-oppression Network. Available at: https://theantioppressionnetwork.com/allyship/. Accessed June 21, 2022.
2. Hamilton A. Allies of the Negro. Opportunity: Journal of Negro Life 1943;21(3):115–7.
3. Word of the year 2021 | Allyship | Dictionary.com. Available at: https://www.dictionary.com/e/word-of-the-year/. Accessed June 21, 2022.
4. Fortune 500 list of companies 2022 | Fortune. Available at: https://fortune.com/fortune500/. Accessed June 21, 2022.
5. Allyship | Rare with google. Available at: https://rare.withgoogle.com/program/allyship-training/. Accessed June 21, 2022.
6. Gompers P, Kovvali S. The other diversity dividend. Harv Bus Rev 2018;96(2):72–7.
7. Mason B, Ross WAJ, Bradford L. Nth dimensions evolution, impact, and recommendations for equity practices in orthopaedics. J Am Acad Orthop Surg 2022;30(8):350–7.
8. Warren MA, Warren MT. The EThIC model of virtue-based allyship development: a new approach to equity and inclusion in organizations. J Business Ethics 2021;1:1.
9. Bourke J, Espedido A. Why inclusive leaders are good for organizations, and how to become one. Harv Bus Rev; 2019. Available at: https://hbr.org/2019/03/why-inclusive-leaders-are-good-for-organizations-and-how-to-become-one. Accessed June 21, 2022.
10. Salter NP, Migliaccio L. Allyship as a Diversity and Inclusion Tool in the Workplace. In: Divers within Divers Management (Advanced Ser Management, Vol. 22), 22. Emerald Publishing Limited; 2019. p. 131–52. https://doi.org/10.1108/S1877-63612019 0000022008.
11. Wolf J., Leadership Strategies: Women in Hand Surgery [video]. Hand.e: American Society for Surgery of the Hand, 2019. Available at: https://www.assh.org/hande/s/watch?id=aBP0a000000LTYXGA4. Accessed September 17, 2022.
12. Galvez M., Dacus A., Bradford P., et al., Diversity and Inclusion: How to be an Antiracist Hand Surgery Educator [video]. Hand.e: American Society for Surgery of the Hand, 2021, Available at: https://www.assh.org/hande/s/watch?id=aBP5b0000008fr1GAA. Accessed September 17, 2022.
13. Adams J. Having It All: Balancing Work and Home Demands of Being a Hand Surgeon [video]. Hand.e: American Society for Surgery of the Hand. November 18, 2019. Accessed September 17, 2022. https://www.assh.org/hande/s/watch?id=aBP0a000000LTYSGA4.
14. About Us. Project Implicit. 2011. Available at: https://implicit.harvard.edu/implicit/aboutus.html. Accessed September 17, 2022.
15. Grova MM, Donohue SJ, Bahnson M, et al. Allyship in surgical residents: evidence for LGBTQ competency training in surgical education. J Surg Res 2021;260:169–76.
16. Rodríguez JE, Campbell KM, Pololi LH. Addressing disparities in academic medicine: what of the minority tax? BMC Med Educ 2015;15(1). https://doi.org/10.1186/S12909-015-0290-9.
17. Williamson T, Goodwin R, Ubel P. Minority Tax Reform — Avoiding Overtaxing Minorities When We Need Them Most. New England Journal of Medicine 2021;384:1877–9.
18. Melaku T, Beeman A, Smith D. Be a Better Ally. Harvard Business Review 2020;98(6):135–9.

Recruitment of the Next Generation of Diverse Hand Surgeons

Claire A. Donnelley, MD, Andrea Halim, MD,
Lisa L. Lattanza, MD, FAOA, FAAOS*

KEYWORDS

• Diversity recruitment • Hand surgery • Pipeline programs

KEY POINTS

- Hand surgery encompasses a diaspora of pathology and patients, yet the surgeons treating this population are not commensurately diverse.
- A physician population that more closely reflects the population it treats consistently leads to improved patient outcomes.
- Although there has been an increase in the diversity of surgeons entering into pipeline specialties such as General Surgery, Plastic Surgery, and Orthopaedic Surgery, the percentage of these trainees lags behind recruitment into other specialties and the overall makeup of practicing hand surgeons remains largely homogenous.
- Pipeline programs beginning as early as high school have been an effective tool to increase the number of surgical trainees entering historically White male dominanted specialties such as Hand Surgery.
- Emphasis on increasing diversity in leadership roles, actively seeking cultural change, and minimizing disincentives toward successful careers in surgical specialties is essential. Passive expectation of increased diversity and cultural change is not enough. Diversity recruitment must be an active process and iterated goal.

INTRODUCTION TO HAND SURGERY

The human hand is a remarkable structure, composed of dense, precise anatomy that works in concert for daily functionality. Comensurate to the diversity of structures within the hand is the spectrum of hand pathology. Hand surgeons restore function after traumatic damage; manage neurovascular compromise, degenerative changes, and inflammatory responses; provide relief from soft tissue contracture; and even perform gender affirmation surgery such as hand feminization.[1] As with the spectrum of pathology, the pathway to Hand Surgery is equally diasporic; hand surgeons come from a diversity of training backgrounds, including Orthopaedic Surgeons, Plastic Surgeons, and General Surgeons with hand fellowship training (**Fig. 1**). Although other specialties have made strides in becoming representative of the patient populations they treat, Hand Surgery lags behind, particularly with the recruitment of women and other historically excluded identities. Organizations such as the Perry Initiative seek to create pipelines to expose women and underrepresented in medicine (UIM) students to Orthopaedic Surgery and form important mentorship networks. Although there remains much work to be done, there are efforts to recruit and retain young women and UIM applicants with the hopes of having a more diverse next generation of hand surgeons.

Department of Orthopaedics and Rehabilitation, Yale University, PO Box 208071, New Haven, CT 06520-8071, USA
* Corresponding author.
E-mail address: lisa.lattanza@yale.edu

Hand Clin 39 (2023) 111–118
https://doi.org/10.1016/j.hcl.2022.08.009

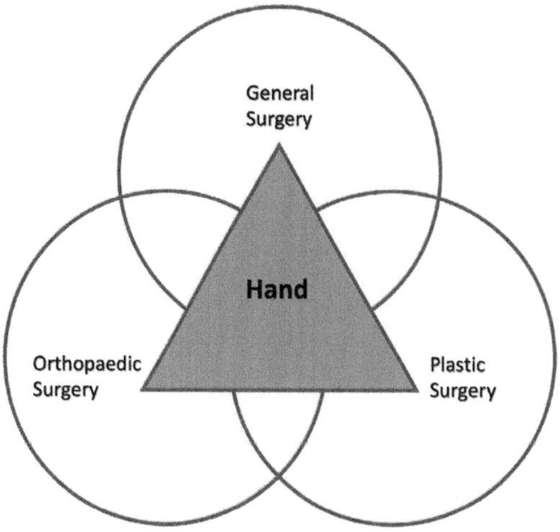

Fig. 1. Hand surgeons derive from multiple specialties: Orthopaedic Surgery, Plastic Surgery, and General Surgery may all develop future hand-specialty surgeons.

Why Does Diversity Among Hand Surgeons Matter?

It is important that the field of surgery be populated by a diverse group of people. Diversity encompasses gender identity, race, ethnicity, training, and lived experiences. There are many reasons why diversity is important. Heterogenous teams demonstrate greater creativity and innovation and consistently outperform homogenous teams when solving problems, performing tasks, and sourcing information.[2] When sourced collaboratively, different backgrounds and experiences lead to better solutions.

Diversity among surgeons is also essential in addressing health disparities.[3,4] Medical treatment may be avoided or delayed due to mistrust of the medical community, remnants of historically exclusionary and unethical practices, underrepresentation, or fear of discrimination.[5,6] Patients who do not share key identities with their treating providers have been shown to receive worse care[3,7] and are less satisfied with their treatment.[8] In addition to representation (or lack thereof) within the medical community, quality and type of health care is modified by factors such as sex assigned at birth, race or ethnicity,[9] socioeconomic status,[10] insurance status, and language proficiency.[5] For example, in one 2016 analysis of more than 13,000 patients, African-Americans and uninsured individuals were significantly less likely to undergo replantation of a traumatic digit amputation than their White, insured counterparts.[11] In cases of upper extremity trauma, uninsured patients are also more likely to be transferred than their insured counterparts, often delaying access to time-sensitive, limb salvage procedures such as revascularization or reimplantation.[12] These disparities continue in nonemergency Hand Surgery. In a 2021 review of carpal tunnel release, older patients and patients with private or workers compensation insurance were more likely to receive surgical intervention, whereas women; patients with Medicare and Medicaid; and patients of Asian, African American, and Hispanic descent were less likely to undergo surgical management.[7] UIM physicians mitegate these inequalities as they facilitate representative of the patients they treat, are more likely to treat uninsured patients, and are more likely to work within underserved communities.[13–16]

Principles of Recruiting Students and Trainees to Hand Surgery

In 1958, there were 10 women board-certified orthopaedic surgeons in the United States.[17] By 2021, with only 1,100[17] women of the nearly 23,000 orthopaedic surgeons in practice, women in Orthopaedic Surgery remain well below the "30% threshold" critical mass to achieve and maintain an ongoing diverse workforce.[17] An even smaller proportion of orthopaedic surgeons identify as a racial or ethnic minority. Only 3% of practicing orthopaedic surgeons identify as Black,[18] and 0.6% of orthopaedic surgeons identify as Black women. Within the field of Hand Surgery, a 2021 review found that of the 614 surgical faculty associated with hand fellowship programs, about 15% are women.[19] Although the percentage of racial, ethnic, and other minorities including Lesbian, Gay, Bisexual, Transgender, Queer, Intersex, Asexual, Allies, and more (LGBTQIA+) hand surgeons are not readily available, open members of these minority communities are rare. Clearly, although strides have been made since 1958, there is still significant work to be done to increase diversity in Hand Surgery.

Currently, the pipeline of women in medical school is equal to that of men, with women representing 56% of undergraduate students and 51% of medical students.[19] Early college performance indicators demonstrate that female high school students are as qualified or more qualified than their male counterparts to pursue science, technology, engineering, and mathematics (STEM) fields such as engineering and Orthopaedics, but this is not seen in practice.[17] This representation seems to break down in the transition from medical school into residency. A 2021 report generated from 15 years of Graduate Medical Education Track data demonstrated that women medical students matching into Orthopaedics lagged behind all other surgical specialties.[20] As of 2012, women represented just less than 20% of Hand Surgery trainees, 17% trainees of Asian descent, 3% trainees of African American descent, and 5% trainees of Hispanic descent.[4] Within the trainee pipeline to Hand Surgery, at 36% and 28%, General Surgery and Plastic Surgery, respectively, have the most women surgical trainees, with Orthopaedic Surgery lagging behind at 14%. Orthopaedic Surgery, in addition, has less ethnic diversity, with 78% Caucasian orthopaedic trainees, compared with 69% Caucasian trainees in Hand Surgery, 72% in Plastic Surgery, and 63% in General Surgery.

To improve diversity in Hand Surgery, more effort must be made to recruit women and UIM into surgical residencies. These recruitment efforts must be made at every step of the training pipeline from high school and beyond, including addressing the recruitment gap of UIM candidates into medical school. As the obstacles to recruiting diasporic individuals into the Hand Surgery pipeline differ at every step of the process, so too must the solutions be tailored to each stage of training.

Pipeline Programs

Lack of early exposure to Orthopaedic Surgery is one of the biggest obstacles to recruitment. Pipeline programs are organizations designed with the goal of increasing diversity by educating and mentoring young people from underrepresented groups. Without such programs, those groups are often at a disadvantage in pursuing fields such as Hand Surgery. For example, men are significantly more likely than women to have exposure to Orthopaedics before medical school.[17] Early intervention (eg, high school) programs seek to mentor young women and UIM students in order to minimize this exposure gap. The long-term goal of pipeline programs is to surpass critical mass diversity thresholds.

Several pipeline programs exist specifically to engage and inspire young people from underrepresented groups to consider specialties in Orthopaedic Surgery. It is important to note that the challenges of attaining diversity are not the same for all groups. Although the number of women has reached and surpassed the number of men in medical school, there is a persistent lack of women choosing surgical specialties, particularly Orthopaedic Surgery. Additionally, there remains adeficit in medical school matriculates of color, men and women. This pipeline problem leads to an even bigger gap with regard to improving diversity in Orthopaedic Surgery and becomes progressively more challenging with the further subspecialized field of Hand Surgery. Depending on where the pipeline to Hand Surgery narrows, different strategies are required.

The Perry Initiative

The Perry Initiative represents one of the most direct and successful methods of creating a pipeline for women to pursue Orthopaedics—and eventually to consider Hand Surgery as a career. This Initiative is named after Dr Jacquelin Perry, who was among the first women certified by the American Board of Orthopaedic Surgery. In 2009 the Perry Initiative, a 501c3 nonprofit organization, was founded by Dr Lisa Lattanza (Orthopaedic Surgeon) and Dr Jenni Buckley (Engineer) with the purpose of recruiting and inspiring high school–aged women to pursue the traditionally male-dominated fields of Orthopaedic Surgery and engineering.[17] The Perry Initiative is composed of several key programs: the Perry Outreach Program (POP) targeted toward high school–aged women, the Medical Student Outreach Program (MSOP) targeted toward women in medical school, and Orthopaedics in Action (OIA) with curriculum for STEM students in middle and high school. As of 2022, more than 14,000 women, graduates of 341 high schools, and 141 medical schools have completed POP and MSOP.[17]

The POP is a hands-on full day course that exposes young women to engineering principles taught through the lens of Orthopaedic Surgery. Activities include simulated saw bone surgeries, suturing, lectures from prominent women orthopaedic surgeons and engineers, and a mentoring program. Approximately 1600 students attend more than 50 programs nationwide annually. The annual career progress of POP alumnae has been tracked with follow-up surveys since 2014. Of 1115 responses (12% response rate), approximately 90% of Perry Initiative Program (POP) alumnae matriculate into STEM majors and 55% note an intention to pursue medicine, with 52.4% noting continued interest in Orthopaedic Surgery.[17] POP programming was cited nearly universally as the impetus for initial and continued interest in Orthopaedic Surgery.

In 2012 MSOP was started for female-identifying or nonbinary first to third year enrolled MD or DO students, now with more than 70 programs annually. MSOP consists of programming that emphasizes hands-on Saw Bones surgical simulations, lectures on careers in Orthopaedic Surgery, work-life balance question/answer sessions, and opportunities for enduring mentorship. Within MSOP participants, the annual match rate into Orthopaedics is 22%. Since its inception,

20% of the women who participated in an MSOP program have gone on to match into an Orthopaedic Surgery residency, compared with 1% of women medical students overall who match into Orthopaedic Surgery. For example, with an overall match rate into Orthopaedic Surgery of 68% in 2021 (1470 applicants with 875 spots), there was a 20% match rate within Perry Initiative graduates, higher than the current percentage of female residents in Orthopaedics.[21] Although the Perry initiative does not specifically recruit women into Hand Surgery, creating a pipeline to directly increase women in Orthopaedics allows for a more diverse pool of future Hand Surgery fellowship applicants.

In 2016, the Perry Initiative created OIA in order to have even a wider reach, which are STEM compliant kits that can be purchased for use in junior high and high school science classes. These kits have now been requested by more than 200 classrooms within the United States.[17] Since 2020, the Perry Virtual Experience and Virtual Medical School Outreach Experience have also been developed and have now reached more than 1800 women in high school, college, and medical school.[17]

Nth Dimensions

The Nth Dimensions Program was founded by Dr Bonnie S. Mason in 2004 as a pipeline program to encourage women and UIM medical students to pursue Orthopaedics. Since its inception, Nth Dimensions has expanded to include recruitment of UIM individuals into many specialties, not just Orthopaedics. The program consists of an 8-week clinical research program between the first and second years of medical school. During this time, students participate in musculoskeletal lectures, practice-based workshops, and research projects and presentations. Mentorship and professional development opportunities derived during this summer continue throughout the remainder of medical school. Between 2005 to 2012, 118 students completed the 8-week clinical and research Nth Dimensions/American Academy of Orthopaedic Surgeons (AAOS) Summer Internship Program.[18] From tracked data, women who completed the internship had increased odds of applying into Orthopaedic Surgery compared with national controls (35% vs 1%, respectively).[18] UIM also had increased odds of applying into Orthopaedic Surgery compared with national controls (31% vs 3%, respectively). Across the 8 years of Orthopaedic summer intern cohorts, the overall match rate of applicants into Orthopaedic Surgery was 76%, which was significantly higher than national controls.[18]

Support/Networking Groups

Many groups and societies exist with the function and purpose of bringing together women and UIM to support and encourage professional success and growth. These groups function as excellent sources of academic support but can also be a place to find advocates against discrimination. Many of these groups also offer pipeline support as part of their programs and initiatives.

The Ruth Jackson Orthopaedic Society

Founded in 1983, the Ruth Jackson Orthopaedic Society (RJOS) serves as a networking and support group for orthopaedic women of all training levels, from high school through established careers. Dr Ruth Jackson was the first practicing female orthopaedic surgeon in the United States. The group offers diverse mentorship opportunities. Workshops are developed and catered to trainees at all levels. For example, during the COVID-19 pandemic, mock virtual interview practice sessions were made available for female medical students applying into Orthopaedics.

The J. Robert Gladden Orthopaedic Society

The J. Robert Gladden Orthopaedic Society (JRGOS) was founded in 1998, named after the first Black orthopaedic surgeon, with a mission to increase diversity within the orthopaedic profession and promote the highest-quality musculoskeletal care for all people. This society offers membership to many training levels, including medical students interested in Orthopaedic Surgery, and to residents, fellows, and physicians already in Orthopaedics. Opportunities for students include mentoring, mock orals, and notifications of grants and scholarship opportunities.

The American Association of Latino Orthopaedic Surgeons

Founded in 2012 by Dr Ramon Jimenez, the American Association of Latino Orthopaedic Surgeons offers mentorship opportunities as early as premedical students. Mentorship may then continue into medical school, residency, and beyond. The organization offers test prep seminars on examinations such as the MCAT and USMLE step 1 and 2 examinations. There are also scholarships and opportunities made available to members targeted toward increasing the number of Latinx individuals within Orthopaedic Surgery.

The International Orthopaedic Diversity Alliance

Founded in 2019, the International Orthopaedic Diversity Alliance (IODA) is a global organization with the 2022–2024 strategic plan including American

Association of Latino Orthopaedic Surgeons with 3 goals: (1) expanding the reach of global diversity efforts; (2) equipping IODA members with knowledge and tools to create and sustain a diverse, inclusive, and equitable environment; and (3) develop a sustainable organization. The organization has free and open membership, providing access to other members in North America, South America, Africa, the Middle East, Europe, Australia, and Asia Pacific.

Black Women Orthopaedic Surgeons

Founded in 2020, the group Black Women Orthopaedic Surgeons (BWOS) has a described mission statement to support and empower Black women orthopaedic surgeons. It targets current orthopaedic residents and beyond with monthly check-ins, big sister/little sister programs, and mentorship opportunities.

Pride Ortho

Founded in 2020 via a virtual happy hour, Pride Ortho promotes mentorship and a sense of belonging for Lesbian, Gay, Bisexual, Transgender, Queer (LGBTQ) orthopaedic surgeons, allies, and patients, with professional development opportunities available throughout all stages of an Orthopaedic Surgery career. The community welcomes all orthopaedic surgeons (gay, straight, trans, or cis) who are committed to increasing LGBTQ representation and community within the field of Orthopaedics.

Women in Orthopaedics Worldwide

Founded in 2021, the Women in Orthopaedics Worldwide (WOW) is a global organization targeted toward the empowerment of women orthopaedic surgeons through the recognition of intersectionality and barriers in the inclusion of women in Orthopaedic Surgery. WOW offers webinars and symposiums, orthopaedic chapters in Africa, Asia, North America, South America, and Europe, analytics such as a "women in Orthopaedics" heatmap, and showcases of women in Orthopaedics such as a compilation timeline beginning in 1919 with Dr Anna Frumina of Ukraine, the first woman orthopaedic surgeon. Membership in WOW is open to everyone.

Orthopaedic Diversity Leadership Consortium

Founded in 2022, the ODLC is a membership organization offering professional development opportunities to improve the effectiveness and sustainability of diversity efforts in health care. They focus on diversity strategy–oriented speaking engagements, personalized coaching, and leadership development workshops. Membership is available to medical students, residents, industry members, human resource and administrative personnel, and practicing physicians.

In addition to the aforementioned organizations, a variety of other initiatives, such as the B.O.N.E.S Initiative,[22] have been developed. Such programs typically use short-term curriculum and mentorship opportunities that emphasize exposure and access to Orthopaedics during medical school. Funding for such initiatives is often addressed via corporate investment and donations (such as from orthopaedic institutions), personal investments, foundation support, and other partnerships such as Project Lead The Way (PLTW).

Deterrents to Entering the Hand Surgery Pipeline

At every education level, involvement of mentors from the next step in training is invaluable[23] to the trainee experience, particularly mentors who may share some of the lived experiences of identity background.[24] Preresidency, mentors provide insight and guidance into the process of becoming a physician. Many students, particularly if they are from socially disadvantaged backgrounds, may have had minimal exposure to or understanding of the process of becoming a doctor and little or no awareness of the different types of medical or surgical practices available. During residency, faculty-to-resident mentorship may include getting residents involved in research, professional societies, support, guidance, and active demonstration of what leadership and the meaningful practice of medicine looks like. Oftentimes existing as the sole individual of a certain identity within a training program, UIM residents may have the lived experience of feeling apart or othered from their residency program or institution, while simultaneously filling hypervisible roles as ambassadors of their race and/or gender.[24]

Mentorship from women and minority mentors at the faculty level is limited for medical students wishing to enter into surgical subspecialties. For UIM medical students finding *any* mentor may be challenging and even more difficult to find a mentor who shares key components of their identity, such as ethnicity or gender identity. One study showed that as few as 35% of medical students identifying as women were able to find a mentor during a surgical rotation, and of those with a mentor, 90% were men.[23] Even if a mentor may be identified, significant discrimination and negative experiences may occur within the training process. A 2018 systematic review of 120 studies examining medical student rationale for surgical specialty selection or selection to not enter into surgery revealed that 68% to 96% of female medical students experience gender discrimination during their surgical experiences.[23] In contrast, male medical students reported significantly less harassment than female medical students, which correlated with greater interest in surgical careers.[23] Further, perceptions developed over time of surgical subspecialties may be additional deterrents. A 2016 survey of female members of the Ruth Jackson Orthopaedic Society found that perceptions of Orthopaedics included the belief that Orthopaedics was too physically strenuous and that along with a "jock fraternity" culture, there was also a lack of appropriate mentorship.[21] These perceptions were included as disincentives to joining the field. Inappropriate mentorship runs the risk of further deterring trainees. A classic example would be having a mentor who, under the guise of helpfulness or caring, suggests that women may wish to pursue less strenuous professions in order to start a family.

Beyond residency, mentorship remains important. Opportunities for advancement for women and UIM continue to lag throughout the career of an orthopaedic surgeon. For example, of 187 orthopaedic surgery residency programs in the United States, only 6 have appointed women chairs, with 4/6 having been appointed within the last 2 years. Diversity in leadership is correlated with diverse recruitment of trainees, and surgical residency programs that lack diversity are less appealing to women and minority medical students,[23] leading to data demonstrating that Orthopaedic Surgery programs train women residents at unequal rates. Although some programs consistently recruit and train women orthopaedic surgeons, others consistently train none and may wish to improve their recruitment.[20] Promoting diverse candidates to program leadership, fellowship leadership, and involvement in societies such as at the American Society for Surgery of the Hand (ASSH) are important steps to providing the continued, ongoing support that surgeons need after successfully navigating the pipeline—by women and minority surgeons continuing to become leaders in the field, the path for future hand surgeons is made clear.

Section Six: The Application Process

Pipeline projects and initiatives are crucial to inspiring and encouraging women and UIM students to apply to medical school and then to surgical specialties. In order for these programs to be successful, the process of applying to medical school, residency, and fellowship must be examined for sources of bias that may preclude successful applications. With data from medicine and outside medicine, gender discrimination in hiring decisions has been well documented via randomized controlled trials, demonstrating that men are more likely than women to be hired despite matched qualifications, men are more likely than women to receive recommendation for advancement, and men are offered higher salaries.[25] Although hiring processes in medicine are typically left up to institutions, groups such as the support and networking groups mentioned earlier as well as national medical societies have the power and ability to affect these processes, minimize bias, and support the future of a more diverse group of surgeons.

Many potential sources of bias exist in application interviews and selection processes. For medical school, residency, and fellowship, many programs rely heavily on letters of recommendation. However, studies have demonstrated that significant differences exist in how applicants are described. A recent study showed that women are more frequently described as being "pleasant" and "flexible," whereas men were more frequently described using their research and initiative.[26] Even in Plastic Surgery where standardized letters of recommendation have become more common, studies show that gender and minority status tend to predict poorer letters.[27] Similar data also exist for applicants to General Surgery residency.[28] To combat this problem, it may be important for schools and programs to consider letters of recommendation as potential sources of bias and not to weight them as heavily as the more unbiased elements of the application, such as transcripts and publications. However, medical school transcripts have been shown to be biased against ethnic minorities,[29] and publications are subject to the ability to identify and access a research mentor, which can vary based on the institution and other factors. Personal statements may also be weighted more strongly when deemed appropriate. Although even these elements of the application may to some extent reflect unequal opportunities or experiences, they give the applicant a chance to represent themselves.

Several strategies exist that can help to limit bias in application processes, including the following:

- Blinding applications to photograph, gender, sex, school of origin, or other potential sources of bias.
- Including secondary reviewers for applications from UIM or female candidates to ensure these candidates receive serious consideration.
- Placing less weight on letters of recommendation, which themselves have been shown to be sources of bias.[26]

- Placing greater weight on factors that have been shown to predict success including female gender, advanced age, military service, and participation in college athletics.
- Ensuring that each applicant interviews with the same faculty in order to decrease subjective variability.
- Asking all interviewers to participate in bias training before application reviews and interviews.[30]

Ultimately, one of the most important considerations for residency, fellowship directors, and department chairs is that increasing diversity among residents, fellows, and attending surgeons must be actively sought if it is to be successful. It cannot be a passive process.

SUMMARY

The importance of taking an active role in furthering the diversity of our field cannot be understated. Diversity does not happen without proactively seeking it out and valuing it. And when diversity is in place, cultural change follows. It is clear that women and minority surgeons still lack opportunities to speak on the national level and are behind their counterparts in opportunities for academic and career advancement. For example, less than 3% of speakers at the Hip and Knee Society over the last 10 years have been women orthopaedic surgeons.[31] Across the board, specialty societies report fewer women in leadership and attaining monetary awards.[32] In order to change culture, create an inclusive society and give women and underrepresented groups a voice; the decision must be made to prioritize diversity.

It is clear that one of the strongest tools we as surgeons have to create a future generation of diverse surgeons is to get involved within the pipeline to our specialty. A multipronged approach to changing the pipeline could include participating in and building opportunities for exposure to surgical specialties, identifying and addressing gaps in education, participating in meaningful mentorship, making use of societies that value and support diverse students and trainees, and shaping institutional cultures that are supportive of women and minority physicians.[18] If we want to have an ASSH meeting full of surgeons from all backgrounds, it is our responsibility to join a committee, volunteer for the Perry Initiative, reach out to a medical student, participate in the residency application process, and advocate for leadership that represents all of us. Meaningful change will only happen when everyone understands the importance of diversity and steps up to be part of the solution.

DISCLOSURE

Drs C.A. Donnelley and Halim have nothing to disclose. Dr L.L. Lattanza is a founding member of and currently serves on the board of directors for the Perry Initiative.

REFERENCES

1. Lee J, Nolan IT, Swanson M, et al. A Review of Hand Feminization and Masculinization Techniques in Gender Affirming Therapy. Aesthet Plast Surg 2021;45(2):589–601.
2. Van Knippenberg D, van Ginkel WP, Homan AC. Diversity mindsets and the performance of diverse teams. Organ Behav Hum Decis Process 2013; 121(2):183–93.
3. Abelson JS, Symer MM, Yeo HL, et al. Surgical time out: Our counts are still short on racial diversity in academic surgery. Am J Surg 2018;215(4):542–8.
4. Bae GH, Lee AW, Park DJ, et al. Ethnic and Gender Diversity in Hand Surgery Trainees. J Hand Surg Am 2015;40(4):790–7.
5. Feroe AG, Hutchinson LE, Miller PE, et al. Knowledge, Attitudes, and Practices in the Orthopaedic Care of Sexual and Gender Minority Youth: A Survey of Two Pediatric Academic Hospitals. Clin Orthop Relat Res 2022;480(7):1–16.
6. Grova MM, Donohue SJ, Bahnson M, et al. Allyship in Surgical Residents: Evidence for LGBTQ Competency Training in Surgical Education. J Surg Res 2021;260:169–76.
7. Brodeur PG, Patel DD, Licht AH, et al. Demographic Disparities amongst Patients Receiving Carpal Tunnel Release: A Retrospective Review of 92,921 Patients. Plast Reconstr Surg - Glob Open 2021; 9(11):E3959.
8. Day MA, Owens JM, Caldwell LS. Breaking Barriers: A Brief Overview of Diversity in Orthopedic Surgery. Iowa Orthop J 2019;39(1):1–5.
9. Amutah C, Greenidge K, Mante A, et al. Misrepresenting Race — The Role of Medical Schools in Propagating Physician Bias. N Engl J Med 2021; 384(9):872–8.
10. Inglesby DC, Okewunmi J, Williams CS, et al. Hand and Upper Extremity Trauma in the Undocumented Immigrant Population in the United States. Plast Reconstr Surg - Glob Open 2022;10(2):E4117.
11. Mahmoudi E, Swiatek PR, Chung KC, et al. Racial Variation in Treatment of Traumatic Finger/Thumb Amputation: A National Comparative Study of Replantation and Revision Amputation. Plast Reconstr Surg 2016;137(3):576e–85e.
12. Wenzinger E, Singh R, Herrera F. Upper extremity injuries seen at a level 1 trauma center: Does insurance status matter? Ann Plast Surg 2018;80(5): 515–8.

13. Xu G, Fields SK, Laine C, et al. The relationship between the race/ethnicity of generalist Physicians and their care for underserved populations. Am J Public Health 1997;87(5):817–22.
14. Marrast LM, Zallman L, Woolhandler S, et al. Minority physicians' role in the care of underserved patients: Diversifying the physicianworkforce may be key in addressing health disparities. JAMA Intern Med 2014;174(2):289–91.
15. Moy E, Bartman BA. Physician Race and Care of Minority and Medically Indigent Patients. JAMA J Am Med Assoc 1995;273(19):1515–20.
16. Komaromy M, Grumbach K, Drake M, et al. The Role of Black and Hispanic Physicians in Providing Health Care for Underserved Populations. N Engl J Med 1996;334(20):1305–10.
17. Buckley J, Dearolf L, Lattanza L. The Perry Initiative: Building the Pipeline for Women in Orthopaedics. J Am Acad Orthop Surg 2022;30(8):358–63.
18. Mason BS, Ross W, Ortega G, et al. Can a Strategic Pipeline Initiative Increase the Number of Women and Underrepresented Minorities in Orthopaedic Surgery? Clin Orthop Relat Res 2016;474(9):1979–85.
19. Grandizio LC, Pavis EJ, Hayes DS, et al. Analysis of Gender Diversity Within Hand Surgery Fellowship Programs. J Hand Surg Am 2021;46(9):772–7.
20. Van Heest AE, Agel J, Samora JB. A 15-year report on the uneven distribution of women in orthopaedic surgery residency training programs in the united states. JBJS Open Access 2021;6(2). https://doi.org/10.2106/JBJS.OA.20.00157.
21. Harbold D, Dearolf L, Buckley J, et al. The Perry Initiative's Impact on Gender Diversity Within Orthopedic Education. Curr Rev Musculoskelet Med 2021; 14(6):429–33.
22. Earp BE, Rozental TD. Expanding the Orthopaedic Pipeline: The B.O.N.E.S. Initiative. J Surg Educ 2020;77(3):704–9.
23. Peel JK, Schlachta CM, Alkhamesi NA. A systematic review of the factors affecting choice of surgery as a career. Can J Surg 2018;61(1):58–67.
24. Roberts SE, Nehemiah A, Butler PD, et al. Mentoring Residents Underrepresented in Medicine: Strategies to Ensure Success. J Surg Educ 2021;78(2): 361–5.
25. Isaac C, Lee B, Carnes M. Interventions that affect gender bias in hiring: A systematic review. Acad Med 2009;84(10):1440–6.
26. Koichopolos J, Ott MC, Maciver AH, et al. Gender-based differences in letters of recommendation in applications for general surgery residency programs in Canada. Can J Surg 2022;65(2):E236–41.
27. Reghunathan M, Carbullido MK, Blum J, et al. Standardized Letters of Recommendation in Plastic Surgery: The Impact of Gender and Race. Plast Reconstr Surg 2022;149(5):1022–31.
28. Sarraf D, Vasiliu V, Imberman B, et al. Use of artificial intelligence for gender bias analysis in letters of recommendation for general surgery residency candidates. Am J Surg 2021;222(6):1051–9.
29. Boatright D, O'Connor PG, Miller J E. Racial Privilege and Medical Student Awards: Addressing Racial Disparities in Alpha Omega Alpha Honor Society Membership. J Gen Intern Med 2020;35(11): 3348–51.
30. Association of American Medical Colleges. Addressing Implicit Bias in Virtual Interviews.; 2020. Available at: https://www.aamc.org/about-us/equity-diversity-inclusion/unconscious-bias-training.
31. Cohen-Rosenblum AR, Bernstein JA, Cipriano CA. Gender Representation in Speaking Roles at the American Association of Hip and Knee Surgeons Annual Meeting: 2012-2019. J Arthroplasty 2021; 36(7):S400–3.
32. Attia AC, Brown SM, Ladd AL, et al. Representation of male and female orthopedic surgeons in specialty societies. Orthopedics 2021;44(5):289–92.

Printed and bound by CPI Group (UK) Ltd, Croydon, CR0 4YY
08/05/2025
01864715-0009